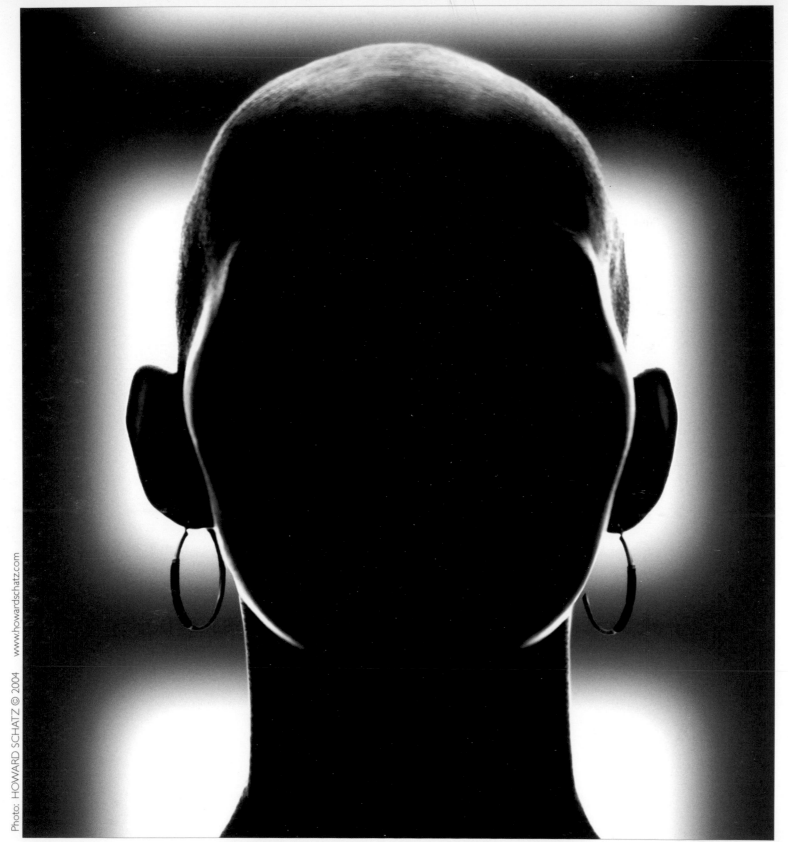

Tamar Bolt #4

TURNING HEADS

PORTRAITS OF GRACE, INSPIRATION, AND POSSIBILITIES

Printed in Singapore

Published by:
Press On Regardless
13636 Ventura Blvd. #422
Sherman Oaks, Ca 91423
USA

A portion of the proceeds of the purchase of this book will go to the American Association for Cancer Research to support cutting edge cancer research. For more information: www.aacrfoundation.org

Library of Congress Cataloging-in-Publication Data
is available from the publisher upon request.
ISBN 13; 978-0-9770074-0-0
ISBN 10; 0-97700740-5

First Edition
Front cover: Harry Langdon 2000
Front cover model: Michelle Davis
Title page: Howard Schatz 2004
Back flap: Harvey Stein 2000

For more information and to order more copies: www.turningheadsthebook.com

For my mother, Louise Strawbridge Hunsicker,
who knew a good bald thing when she saw
one – my father, John Freedley Hunsicker.

And for all these brave women and generous photographers.

FOREWORD

I don't know how we got here or who is to blame. And, I don't know how to get out of it, but women today are never satisfied with how they look.

Either we think we're too tall, too thin, too flabby or fat. If our hair is curly, we want it straight. If it is straight, we want it curly. We're constantly searching for ways to improve. No one looks in the mirror and says, Wow, you couldn't be any better looking.

If that's how we feel about ourselves when we're well, what happens when we're sick? What happens when we get cancer and lose our hair while undergoing aggressive treatment?

It can be devastating.

When I was diagnosed with Stage Two breast cancer, my initial reaction wasn't, Oh my God, I have cancer, I might die; it was, Oh my God, I have cancer, I'm going to lose my hair and then I'll be walking around looking like one of *those* people.

According to the American Cancer Society, 662,000 women get some form of cancer each year. A majority of them will lose their hair while undergoing treatment. As baby boomers age, that number will grow. Think of it. Hundreds of thousands of women a year will have to go through this much-dreaded physical transformation and have their self-image stripped from them.

In a perfect world, we shouldn't feel ashamed of the way we look while fighting cancer; we shouldn't want to hide. We should feel like who we are: beautiful in a different way and more beautiful than ever. But this world isn't perfect. How we currently perceive the disease, how we shrink away from it, requires an attitude adjustment – for the patient, for the people who love that patient, and for the rest of us.

And it's not going to be as hard as you think. All you have to do is look at these pictures and think about what they mean and, inch by inch, you will help change the world with us.

J.S.H. 2006

TABLE OF CONTENTS

FOREWORD BY JACKSON HUNSICKER ~~~~~~~~~~~~~~~ PAGE 6

PORTRAITS ~~~~~~~~~~~~~~~~~~~~~~~~~~~~~~~~~~ PAGE 8

AFTERWORD ~~~~~~~~~~~~~~~~~~~~~~~~~~~~~~~ PAGE 126

ABOUT THE PHOTOGRAPHERS ~~~~~~~~~~~~~~~~~ PAGE 127

THE GOOD & THE GREAT ~~~~~~~~~~~~~~~~~~~~~ PAGE 142

PHOTO CREDITS ~~~~~~~~~~~~~~~~~~~~~~~~~~~ PAGE 144

DOLORES CHAVEZ
age 59, longshoreman

"I have a wonderful support group in my family. We're all longshoremen. My husband, my two sons, two daughters, my brother. They're unbelievable. But it's a roller coaster. Most of the time, we joke about it. It's how we get through the tough times. You need to laugh. When you laugh, you relieve some of the tension you have. Cancer isn't easy, but it's what I have and it's who I am right now.

I have my crying days, too. Those days, I tell myself, Okay, Dolores, you're going to cry today but you only have an hour. Sometimes I can't do it in an hour so I say, Okay, Dolores, you have half the day then go on, get up and go on from there.

That's the roller coaster of it. The good and bad days. But didn't we have those same kinds of days before we got cancer?"

photograph by Stephanie Ellis

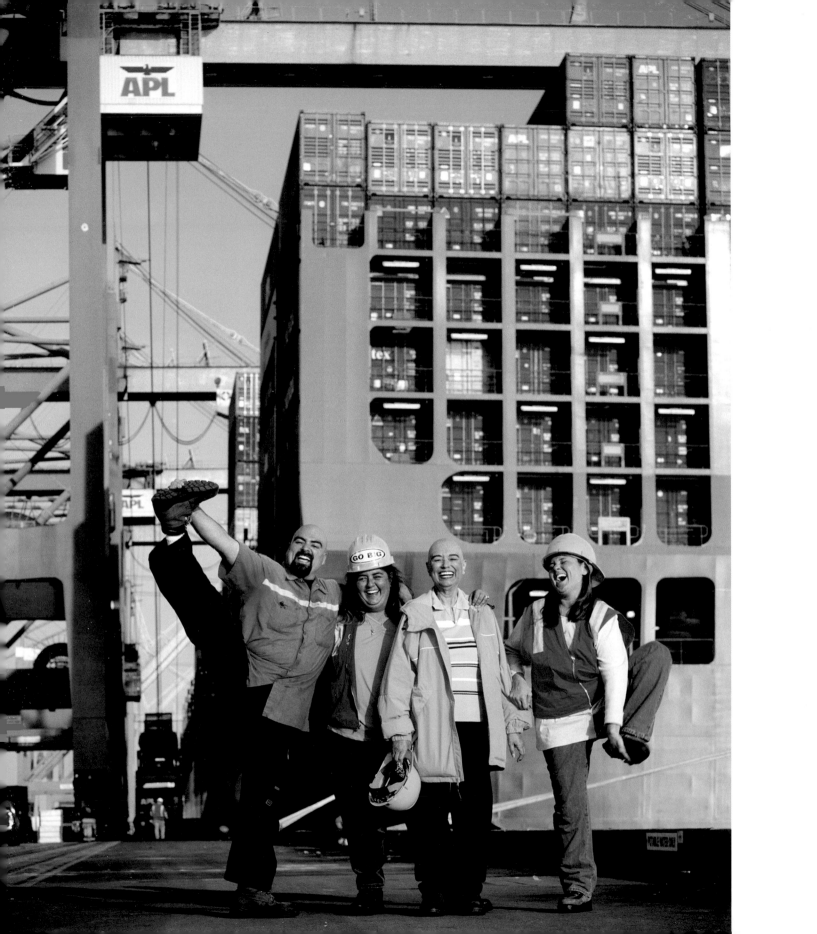

CECILIA PERSSON
age 29, student

"It's awful to lose your hair but you must set it in its proper perspective. I cannot allow it to be important. It's a hassle. You stand out. You wonder if people will be offended. It takes away the choice of whether or not you want to proclaim that you're going through something difficult. Maybe it's like being in a wheelchair – you enter a room and you don't choose if you want to tell someone what you're going through. It's a marker. 'Look at my bald head.' But in the greater perspective of things, I cannot allow any of it to be important.

Losing my hair in comparison to losing my leg was really not that big of a deal. I remember feeling not offended but misunderstood when my friends would say, 'Oh how awful for you to lose your hair. You must be so strong to deal with that.' I remember thinking if you had any idea what I've lost, you wouldn't think that losing my hair was important.

At the end of the day, it is the goodness of your heart that truly matters, not your looks. Not whether you're smart or funny. When you don't have these outer layers you need to feel that you deserve to be loved for who you are. The main thing is that I'm valued as a human being."

photograph by Lauren Greenfield –VII

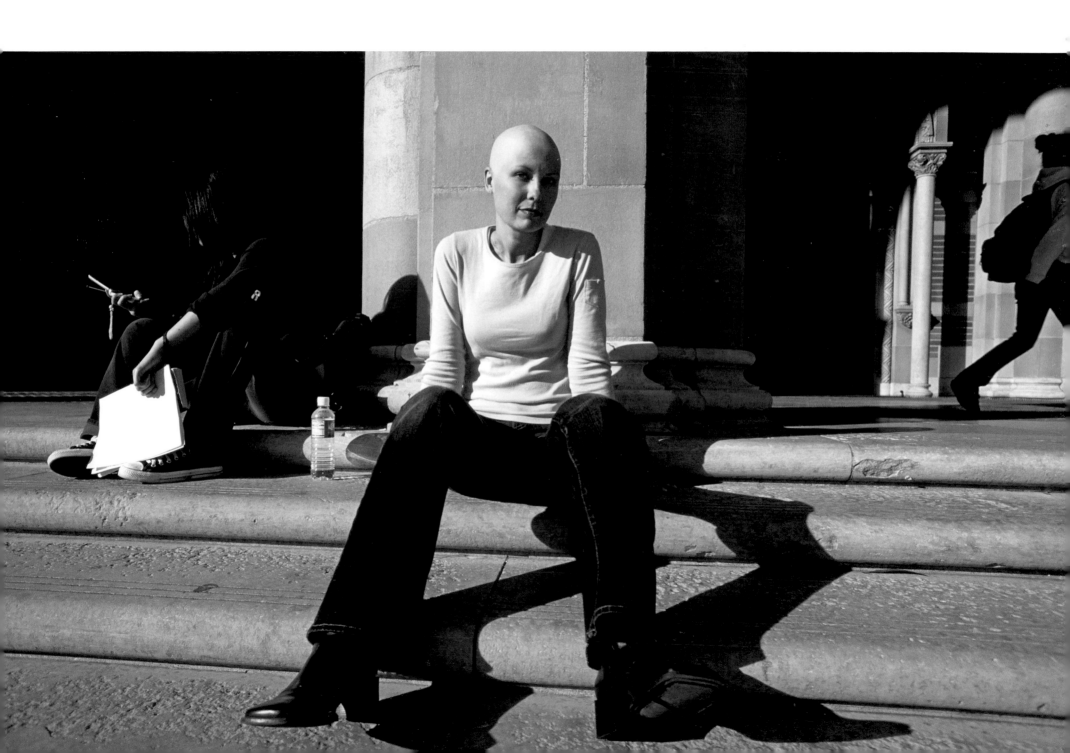

LYDIA SAMUEL
age 45, massage therapist / yoga instructor

"It felt very liberating to have my picture taken without any clothes. I felt like I was being celebrated beauty-wise, even with no hair.

Looking back, I guess the scariest part was when I was about to lose my hair because losing hair or not having it is always associated with shame or punishment or something like that. Once I decided to buzz it off, I was fine. I felt as if I could go on and continue with it and get it over with so I could get back to normal as soon as possible.

I would have liked to have had more knowledge about what cancer was and what the treatments were. I knew nothing. I didn't even know what an oncologist was but then I started educating myself and things became clearer. Just get the best treatment possible and you'll get back to normal and it'll be sweeter at the other end."

photograph by Kevin Lynch

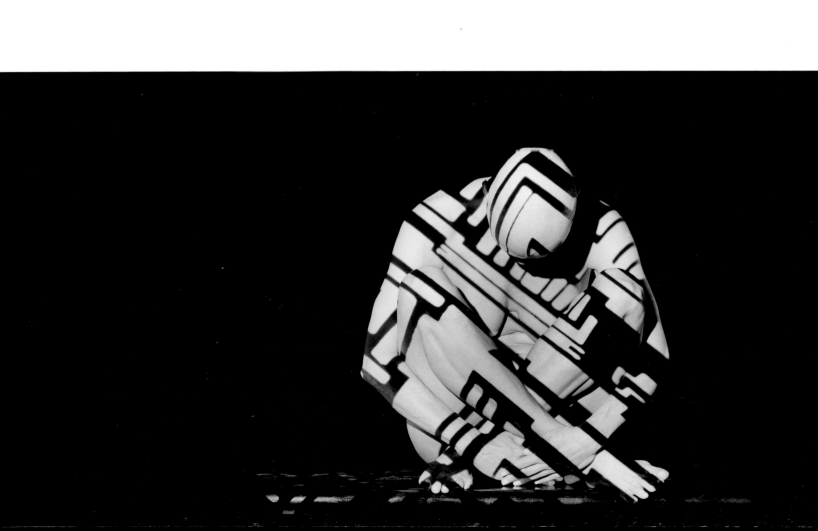

ANGELIA JACKSON
age 49, dental assistant

"It's a day-to-day process. You still wonder, why did I get it? Did I have too much coffee? Did I have too many chocolates? Too much wine? You think something must have caused you to get it. I always had everything checked once a year on my birthday and here I am!

There's been a lot of love and support. My brother and dad call me every morning to ask if I'm okay. My sister lives right next door and my son always asks, 'Mom, you okay?' And then in the night they all call again and ask, 'How you feelin'?' And I answer, 'So far, everything's still working.' We tell each other we love each other and then we go to sleep. They just want to spoil me and I let them."

photograph by Nick Vedros

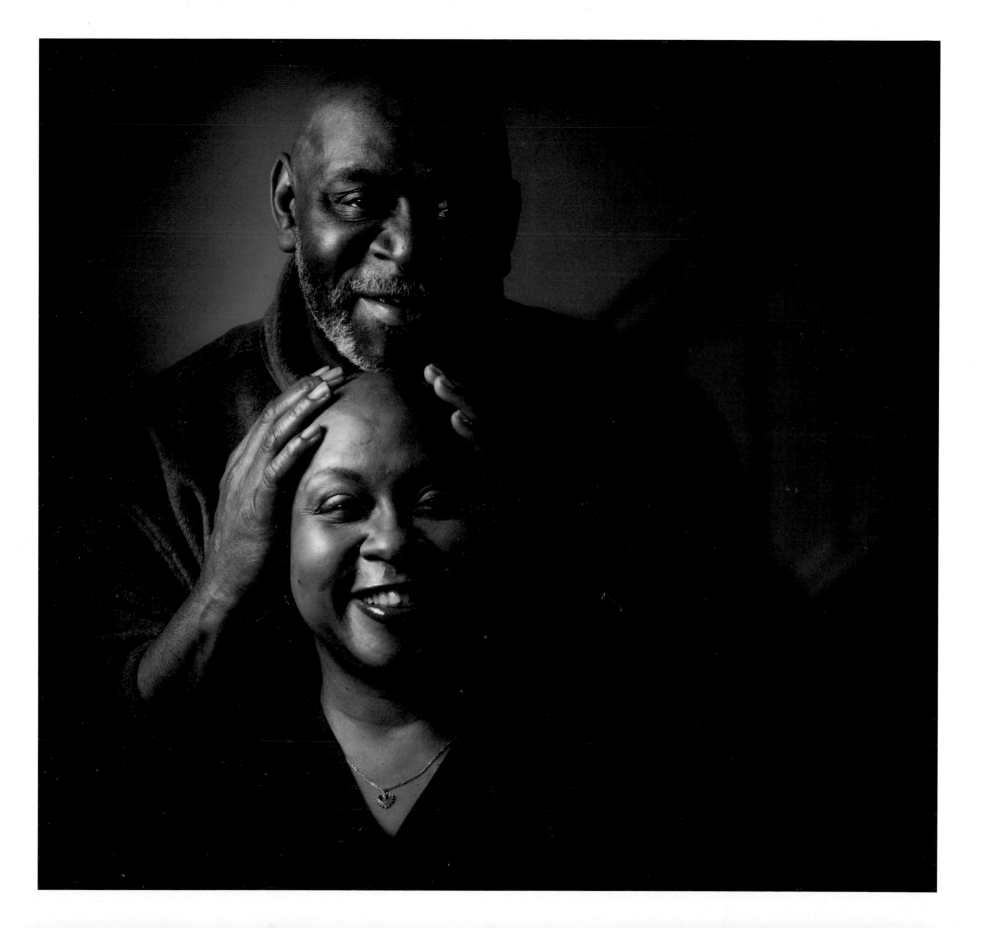

BECKY McINTYRE-PACHECO
age 51, administrative assistant

"When my son was called up to go to war, I said I'd take care of his children but then I got diagnosed. He was worried about me. He didn't want to impose on me while I was sick and I told him, 'I'll fight my battle and you fight your battle and everything will be fine. Don't worry about your children because they're going to be part of my healing.' Children are so open and so wonderful. They've been very positive about it. And so we've all come through it.

I ask myself what is it I would change in my life and I say, Nothing. I'm very blunt and very open and I speak the truth. I stand for what's right. I love people just as they are. I don't expect them to be any different then they are. Life isn't about how much money you can accumulate, rather it's about how much living you can get out of life.

I want to live till I die!"

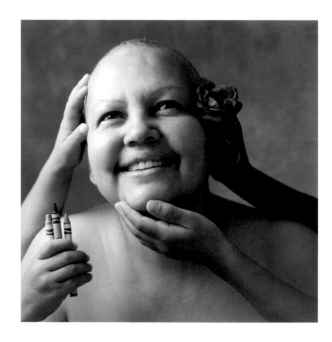

photographs by Karen Kuehn

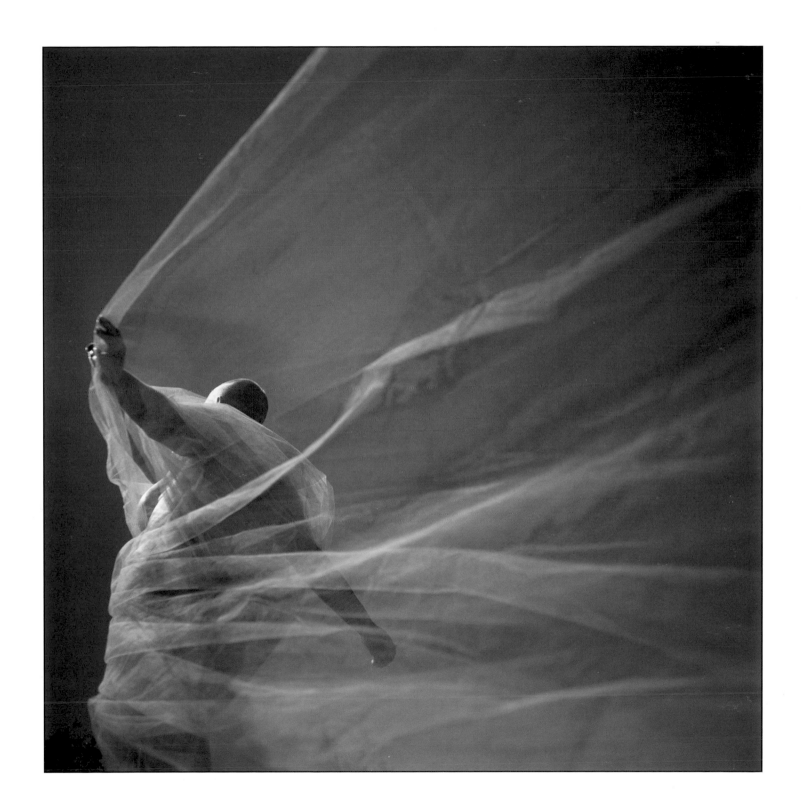

LIDIA SING DE MARTINEZ
age 37, mother / part-time insurance broker

"I know everyone's name who's helping me. Every technician's name. All the nurses and radiologists. I see them as my second family. I look forward to seeing these guys. I put my hope in their hands. I bring them presents, lemon pies, a homemade cake. I think they appreciate it. I think they should be recognized for their work.

I want to make some huge changes in my life. I want to leave my job. I want to take some quality time with my husband and children. You know, it's the small things that are important. Like having dinner together. I even bought place mats and asked my cousin to embroider them with my children's names and Mama and Papa. I like the small things."

photograph by Annie Wells

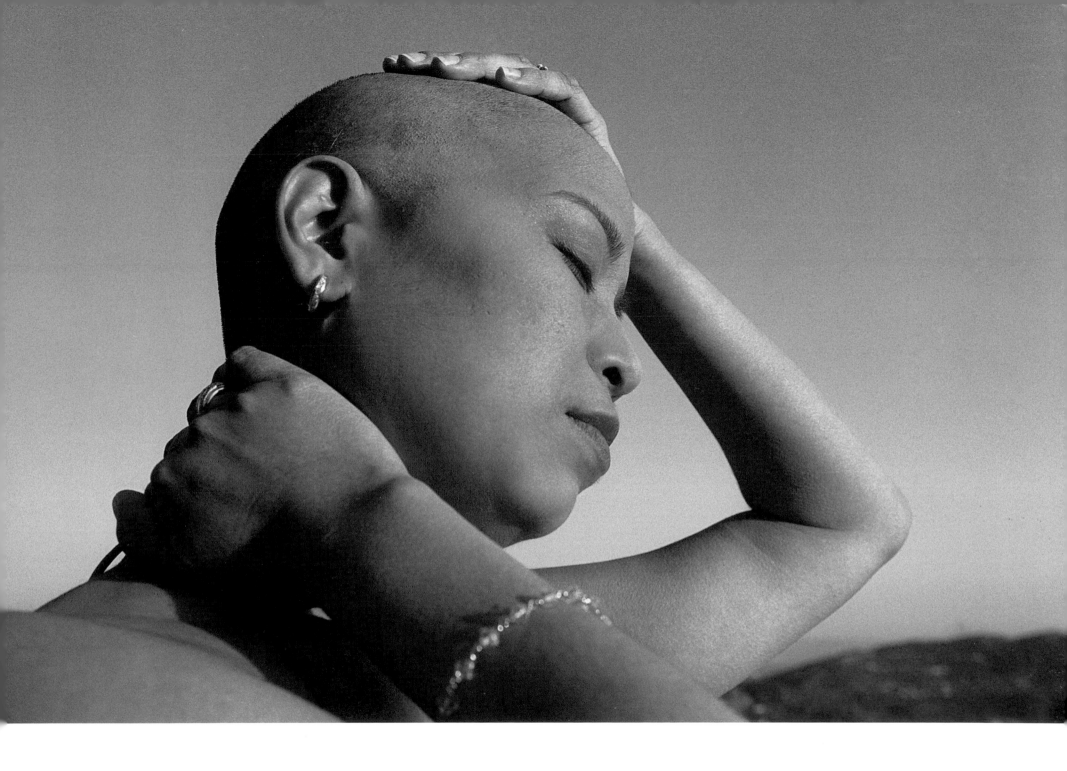

MELISSA ETHERIDGE

age 43, rock n' roll singer / songwriter

"When the Grammys called and asked if I would come I thought, Naaah, I'll just be that bald girl there. But then I found out they wanted me to perform Janis Joplin. I love Joplin. She was a huge inspiration to me and I knew if anyone else were to sing her songs while I was at home watching TV, I'd be cranky. So I said I'd go.

I also knew I'd be far enough away from my last treatment that I'd have enough energy in me to sing a two-minute song. Then I started to wonder if my hair would grow back by then. Would I have a little hair? None? What was I going to have? As the Grammys got closer, I began to think that maybe I should wear a bandanna. I'm just not a wig person, I don't think I could have worn one comfortably. I would have been doing it for other people, not for me. Then I began to wonder if I was going to be afraid of what people would think when they saw me. I didn't want them to think I was sick. Usually a bald head on a woman means she's sick and I didn't want that but then again there was no other option for me.

My stylist found me that jacket. It had a nice high collar and it made my head look grand! So I thought, Okay, I'll go to the Grammys bald! People already knew I had breast cancer. Why not? I'm all about the truth. It felt good that night. I was so cool under the hot lights. It felt great. And my goodness, I was overwhelmed by the response from it. If we can inspire anyone, I say, great – go ahead, be bald, it's sexy!

Now when I see photographs of myself with hair, I think Gosh, so much of my face is hidden. And the energy you feel when you don't have anything on your head! All the energy just goes 'whoosh' – it's right there and there's so much clarity to life bald!"

photograph by Robert Gauthier

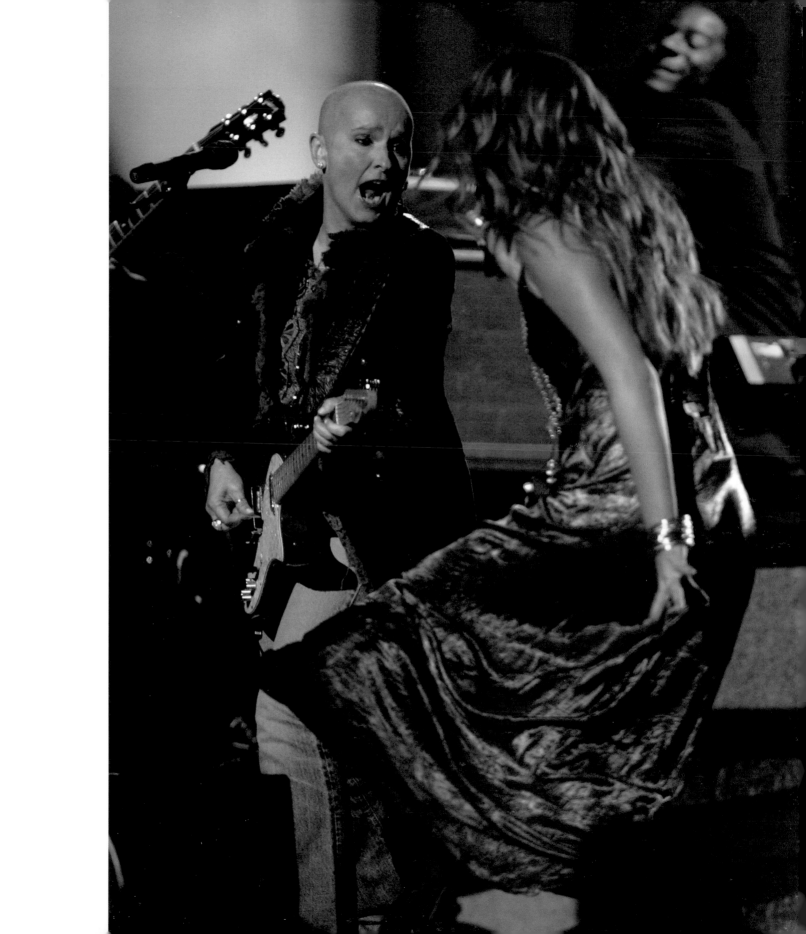

CECELIA DOHERTY
age 48, homemaker / electrician

"Learning to live through adversity is what life is about. I mean, bad things happen to good people through no fault of their own. Going through treatment, I chose to be a positive image to my seven-year-old daughter. As she experiences life's ups and downs, I want her to be able to go through it all gracefully. Dealing with my treatment shows her how to get information, get facts, be conscientious about choosing health-care specialists, work the plan and plan the work and what you have to do, do it!

I can get through this just like my daughter can get through her multiplication tables, one number at a time."

photograph by Rusty Kennedy

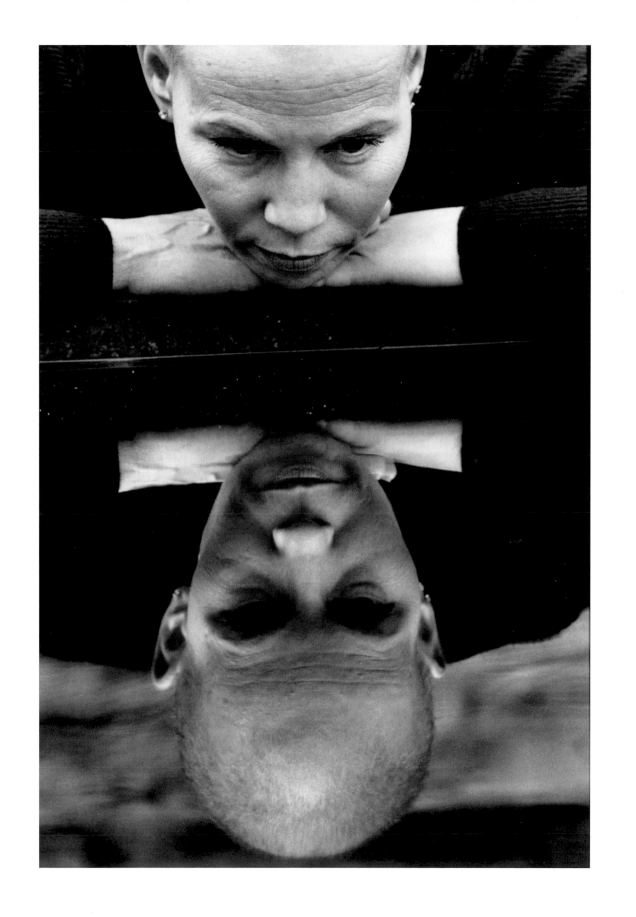

MIMI MORIN
age 62, volunteer worker

"You need a team behind you. (I had my husband and daughter and son-in-law.) They can help you figure out where you are going, what avenue you should take and how you're going to see that rainbow at the end of your journey. It was the first time I wasn't in control over anything and I must say it came out very well.

During treatment, I got much closer to my husband. He knows how much I like to play golf so we started to go golfing together which was good therapy. We had a great time. Most of the time, Mike won. He's better than I am. But don't forget he has a big swing and I'm not a big girl."

photograph by Kenn Long

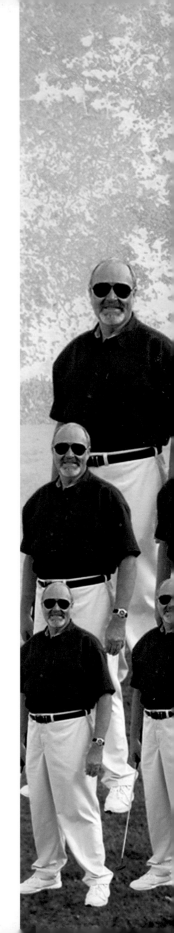

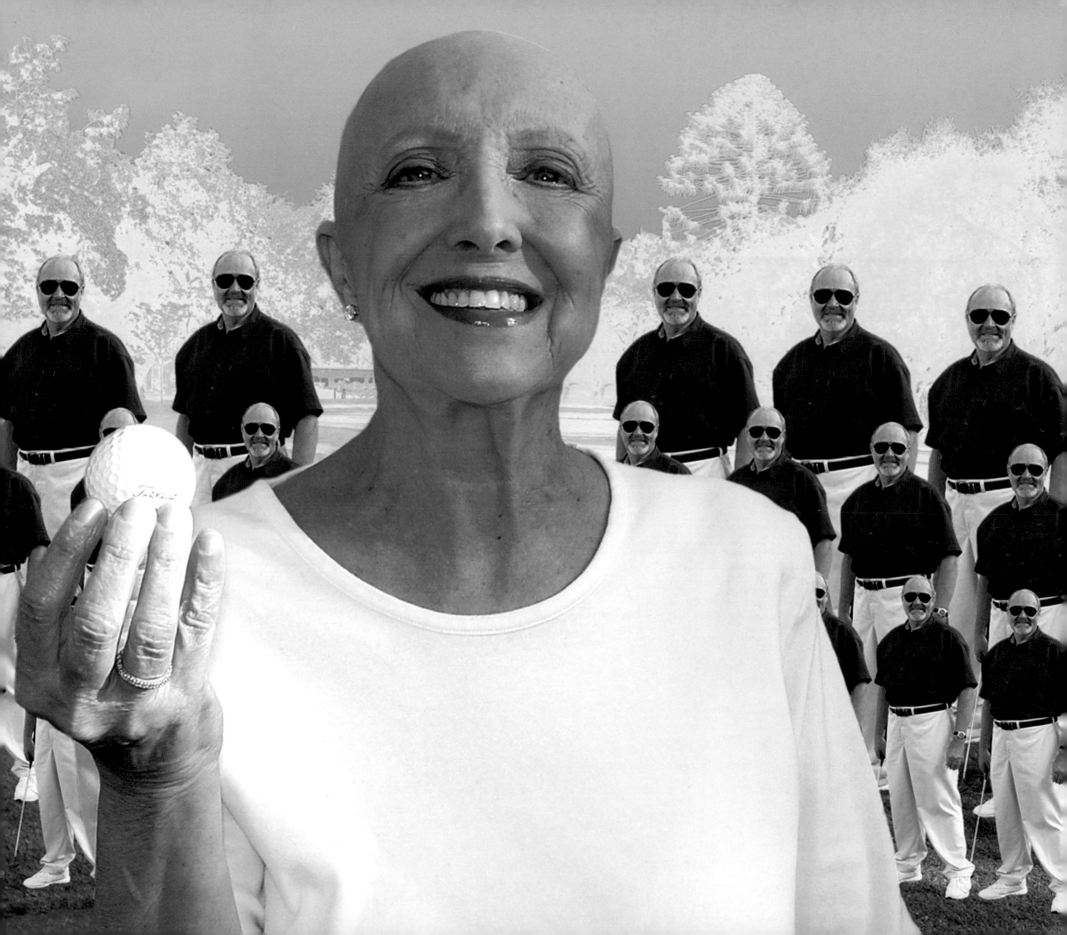

ZOË MORSETTE
age 53, theatrical crafts artist

"At home I put music on in my living room and there's a mirror there and I love to just dance in front of it. Dancing always makes me happy. It makes me feel much more alive.

The visual line is everything in dance. By the visual line I mean how extended your body is. The visual line should be continuous. When you extend your arm, you don't want the hand to hang like a dishrag at the end because it drops the line short. But if you extend the hand, the energy just keeps going out to the end of your fingertips. That way peoples' eyes keep following that extension out. When the head doesn't have any hair on it, like mine doesn't now, this continuous line goes up around my neck and then goes into the curve of my skull without anything interfering with it. It is beautiful. It's so aesthetically pleasing to make lines and shapes with your body. When you do things that give you pleasure, it is easy to forget about the illness and just focus on the joy of the moment."

photograph by Lois Greenfield

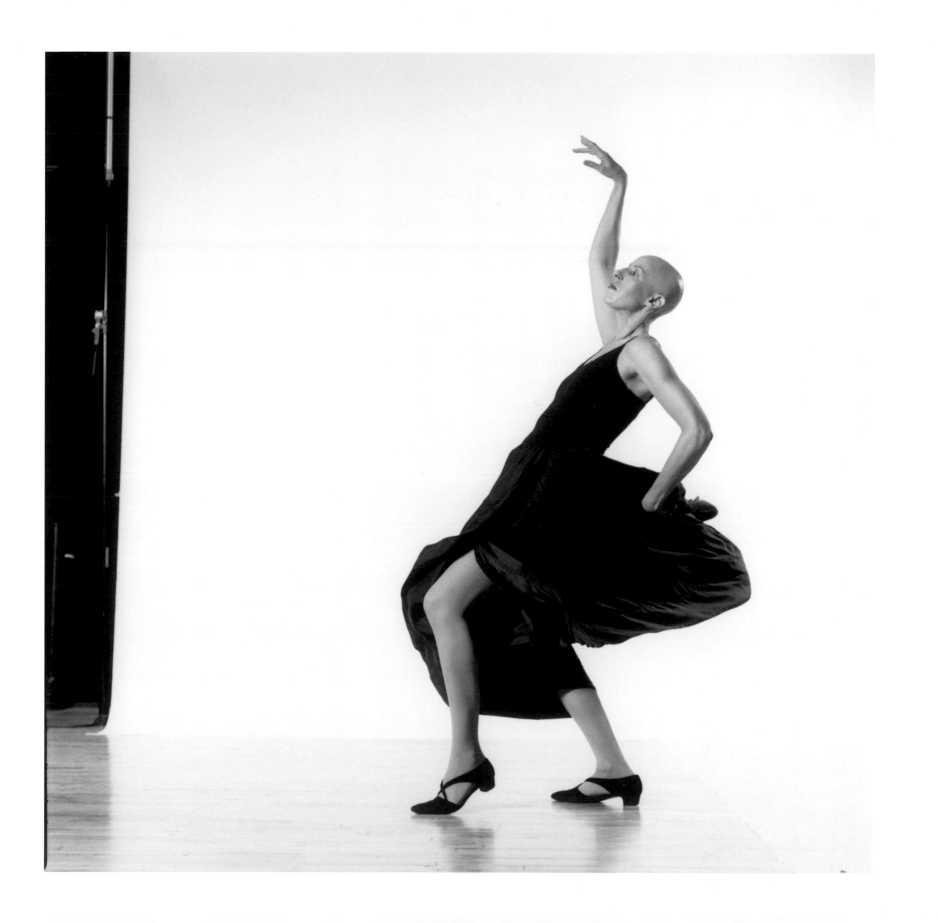

DIKLA BENZEEVI and Jennifer Huang, seated, (see page 94)
age 32, executive assistant

"Before we took this photograph, I'd never been out bald before in public. It felt good not to have a wig. It was warm and it was summer and you felt free and relaxed. We were at Venice Beach in California and there are so many weirdos there that I wasn't self-conscious. We just walked around – Jennifer Huang, David Kennerly and myself – and people would glance at us and then move on.

I'm really close to my family, my three brothers and my relatives in Israel. They have all been extremely supportive. I read a card once that said 'Kindness sprouts lush gardens.' People around me have shown such great support and kindness and love, I hope to tend that ever-growing, nurturing garden for the rest of my life. "

photograph by David Hume Kennerly

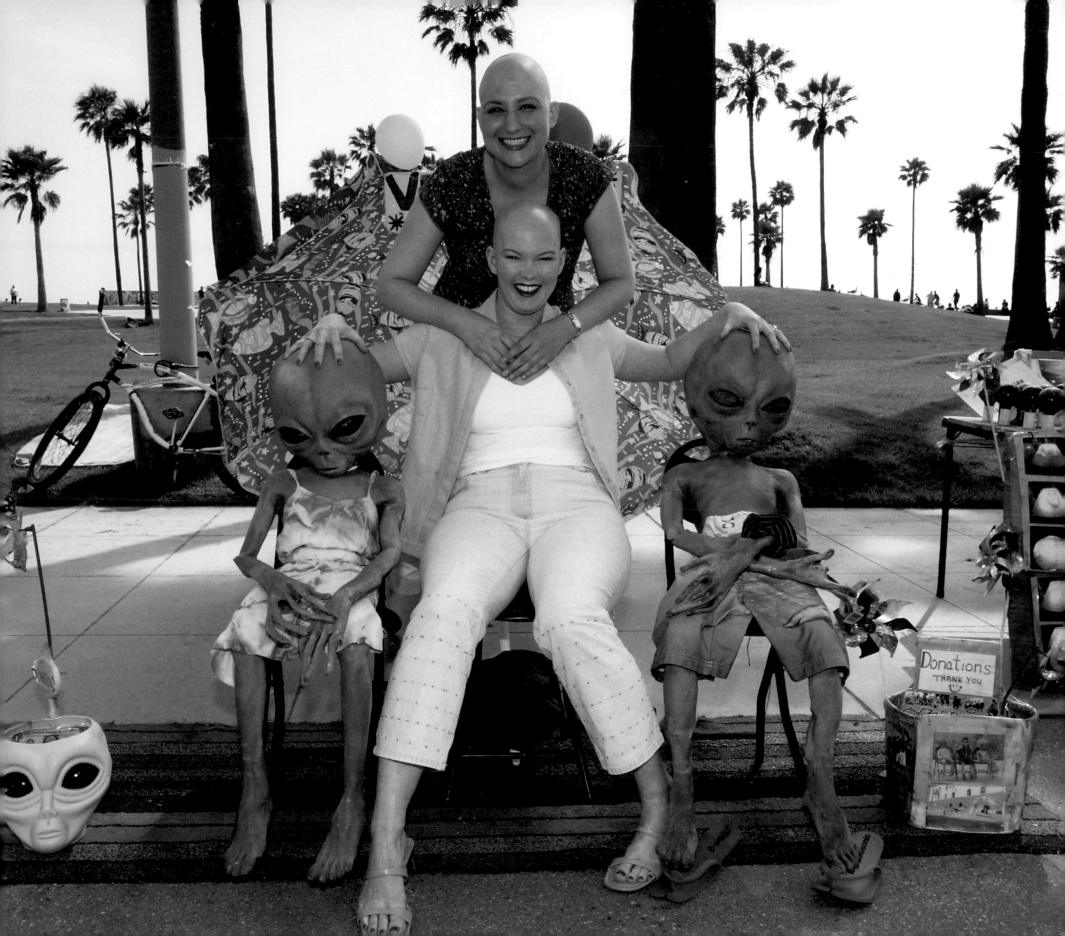

ELIZABETH ARMSTRONG

age 49, museum curator

"I was hoping I would feel okay about going around in public without hair. I'm sorry to say that I found it too difficult. But during my year of baldness, I noticed how many men are choosing to shave their heads. Michael Jordan helped popularize the look in the 1980s, but it has only been in the past few years that a growing and increasingly diverse population of shaved heads has taken to the streets. Today, a bald head can give men a newfound look of power. It is a great equalizer, minimizing surface differences between race, age, and background. Baldness has gone from being a geek look to being a cool look. And if that can be true for men, there's no reason why it can't be true for women.

Once I got over the shock of it, I loved the feeling of being nearly bald, and now I'm not ready to give it up. My closely cropped head feels great underwater, dries in an instant and always looks neat. And, suddenly, I have a liberating new hairstyle that is admired by many people who might not have noticed otherwise. My hope is that more and more women will be comfortable with this look, whether it's chosen or not. Notions of beauty change over time, and baldness has been considered beautiful at different moments throughout history. What better time than now?"

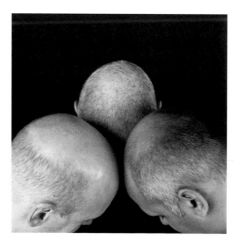

photograph by Catherine Opie

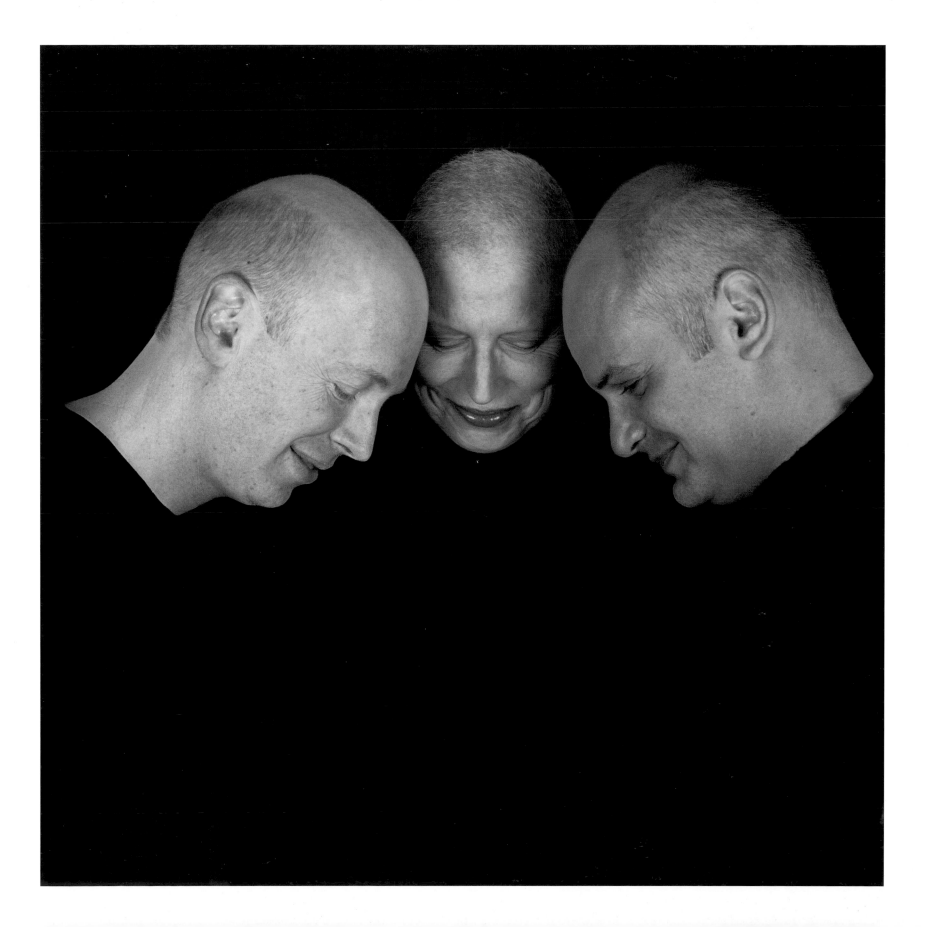

ALICE DEAKINS
age 65, professor of english

"Because I'm an English professor, I looked through a lot of poems about spring. That's when I went through treatment, in the spring, and I was hoping to access its energy. I found the opening piece of Chaucer's *Canterbury Tales*. I realized it was capturing so much of my individual experience.

Chaucer's Prologue talks about people coming together in springtime and going on pilgrimages and going to faraway places, in particular, to holy lands and holy places. That's how I felt, like I was in a faraway land, a distant place. And the idea of a holy place helped me see that all these medical encounters I was in were taking place in a space that was given over to healing.

The pilgrim's goal is to seek healing or to acknowledge someone who has helped you when you're sick. I tried to take this image with me. It gave me a new way of looking at what was happening to me. The places I was going and the people I was meeting were my helpers on this pilgrimage.

Besides, you can't go back. You have to be brave. You meet people you wouldn't have met before and that's always wonderful. You tell your stories – how you're feeling, what happened to you and you help each other out, just like in the *Canterbury Tales*."

photograph by Katy Grannan

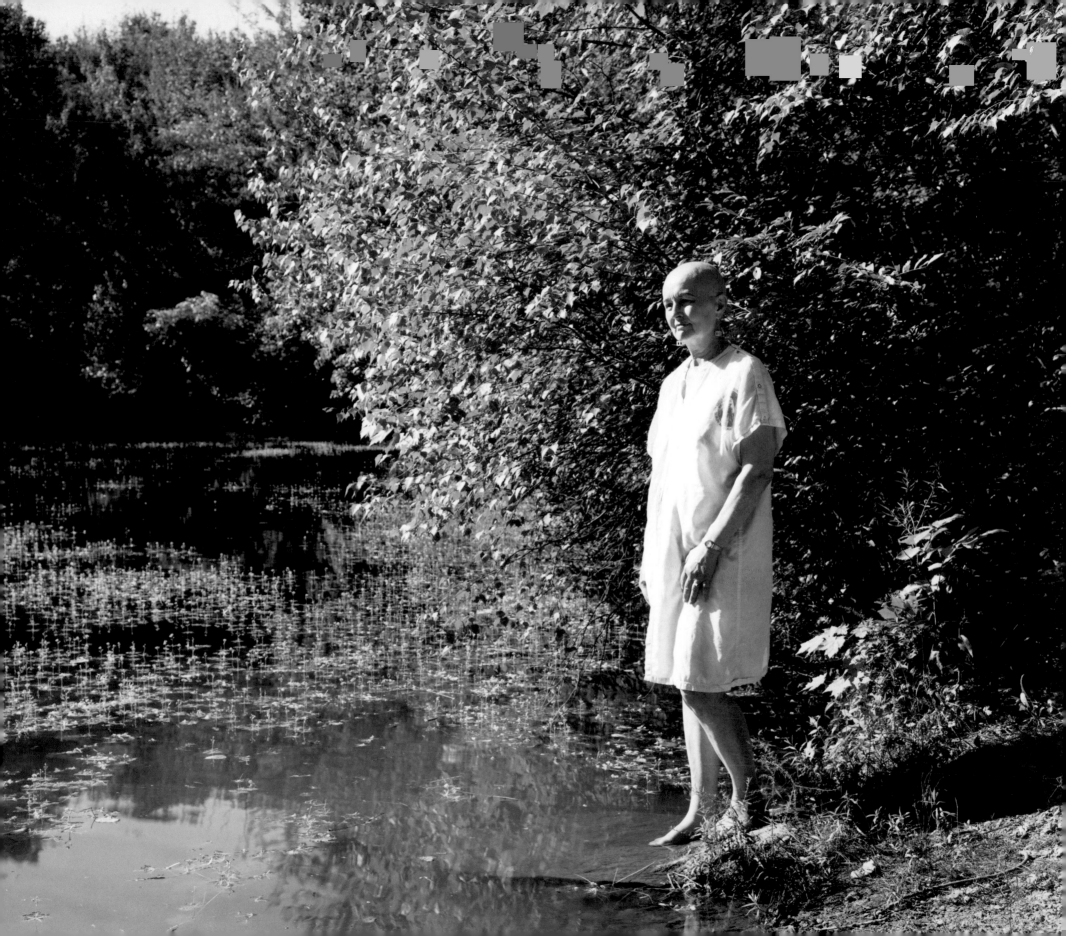

HEATHER HIMELWRIGHT
age 32, insurance broker

"I don't have kids, I have a good marriage. I've got family and fabulous friends and a wonderful support system, but if I had looked back on my life seven months ago, I would have said that I hadn't done very much with my life.

This disease has given me a second chance. It's helped me understand that that's not true, that I have done a lot. I've reached a lot of people and I've probably changed lives in a very, very, very small way because every person you've touched is someone you've changed. I don't care if it's with a smile or a thank-you, whatever the case may be, I have changed lives. We all have.

That's what's really cool about this disease. I've been given this opportunity. Now I can re-commit. I'm going to go out there and touch more people than I ever thought I could. It's going to be an amazing 50 more years. And think what I'll be able to teach my children!

There's a line from *The Last Samurai* that says you see life in every glass of tea, every sip you take, every breath you breathe, you see life. And it's true. I am happy. I'm happy to wake up in the morning. I'm happy to drink that tea. That tea is really, really good. I can breathe life."

photograph by Tom Atwood

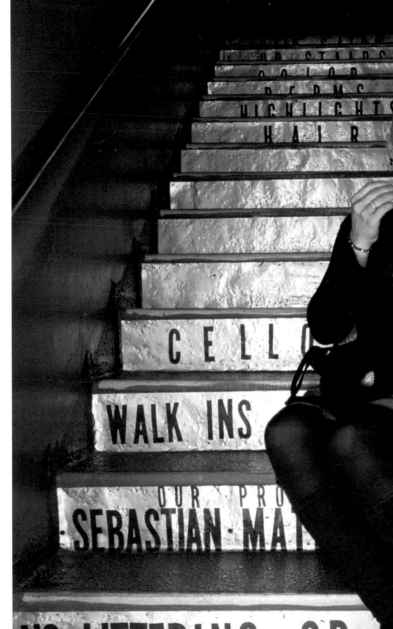

ADELL CARR
age 71, retired hospital administrator

"The first time I lost my hair, the crew in the infusion area said that in fourteen days my hair would go away and in fourteen days it did. I was in the shower and I came out with a towel around my head and my head felt kind of funny. When I took the towel off, there was all this white hair falling all around me.

I went out of the house onto the deck and leaned over the railing and scrubbed my head and my hair just floated away on a very gentle southwest breeze. I thought it was nice because at that point it was spring in Cape Cod and all the birds were building their nests. My silver white hair would be woven into their nests. It was very comforting."

photograph by Sasha

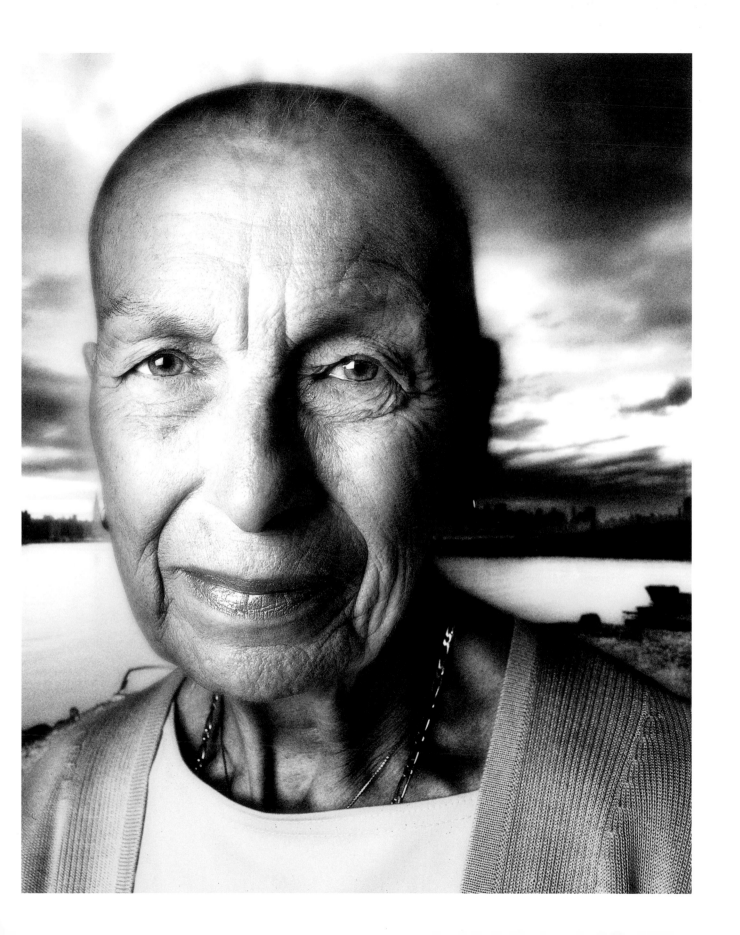

PAM BERTINO
age 57, harley rider

"You have to have fun. You have to laugh. When the negative comes, you have to throw it out.

One of the best things for me? To get on the bike and go. When you're on the bike, you still feel normal. You don't feel sick. It's a fun, free thing. I ride my Harley with my husband and his friends and my girlfriends. And because I'm bald, everyone else gets helmet head but I don't. That's a benefit."

photograph by Ethan Kaminsky

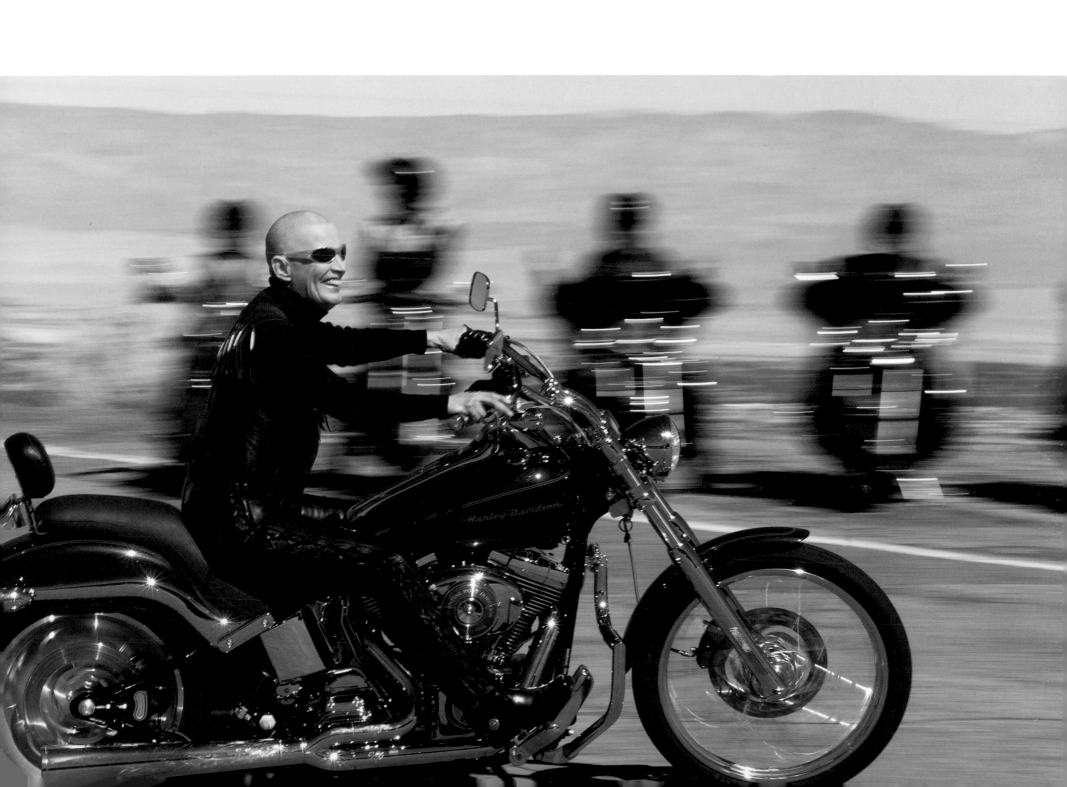

IRENE McKAY
age 43, medical assistant

"At one point during treatment, I didn't want to live anymore. It was really a struggle for me. I remember one day I had all the lights off in the house and I was crying and crying and I prayed to God to take me but then I thought about my son. Who would take care of him? Who would see to his needs? The feeling passed but that was the lowest I'd ever been. There always is a better day. I'm finished treatment, my hair is growing back, my self-esteem is getting better. There is a better, brighter day, you just need to wait."

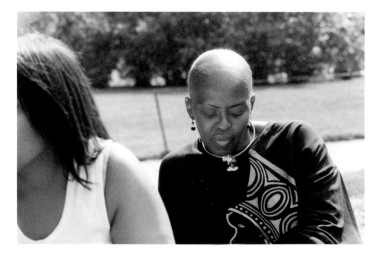

photograph by Amber Amsterdam

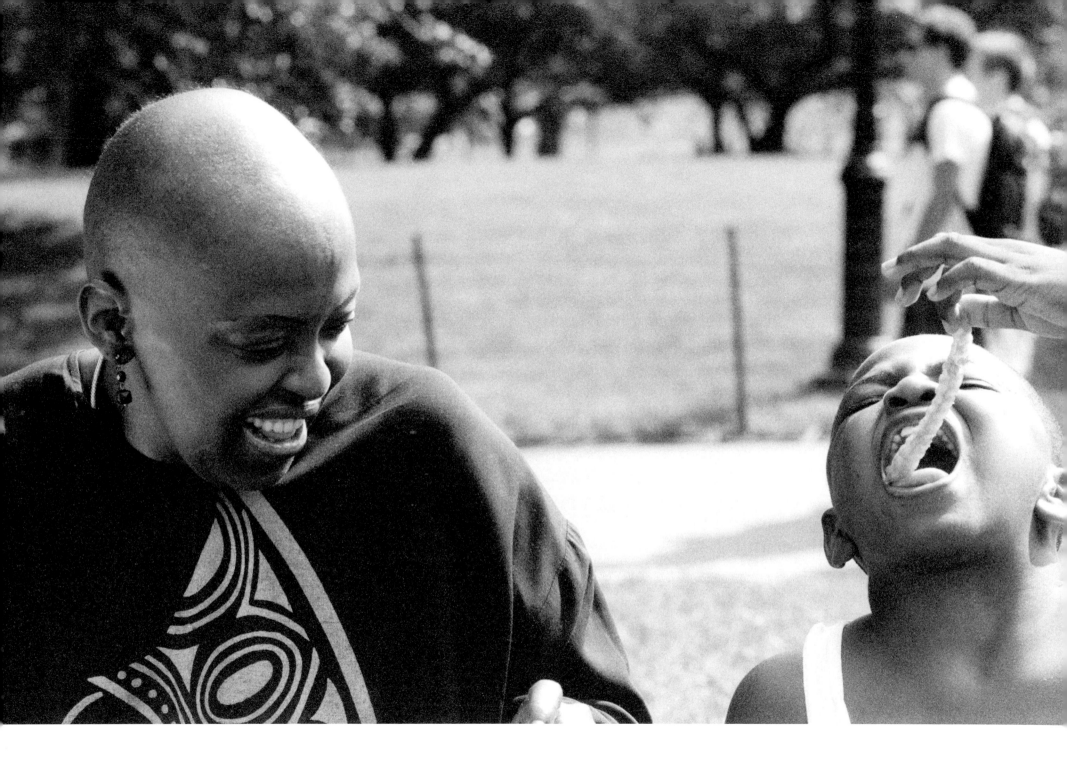

HELEN STEIN

age 58, clinical psychologist / volunteer at Wave Hill, New York

"The day we took this photograph, I met with Clay McBride, the photographer and Craig Cartwright, the painter, at Wave Hill and we walked around the greenhouse and gardens looking for flowers that appealed to us and came upon some magnificent morning glories. We snitched a blossom and went to a room where Craig began painting. The paintbrush felt cool and good on my head. It took about an hour and forty-five minutes. When it was done, we walked over to the greenhouse. Some school kids were visiting the place and one said, 'Look at that cool tattoo!' which is much nicer than 'Look at that bald lady' which is what I thought they might say. Craig started shooting. He took pictures of Marie, the gardener who tends the tropical green house and me together. I had a chance to show my painted head to all the other gardeners there and they loved it.

After the shoot, I planned to catch a train to Washington, DC to visit my sister. I decided not to rub off the painting. I didn't really look for people's reactions at Penn Station or on the train, but I did notice that the seat next to me was probably the last one in the car to be filled. I suspect people didn't know what to think, but I really didn't care, and could see some advantages to my apparently off-putting appearance. When I got to DC and saw my sister, she started laughing. My 7-year-old great nephew, Ian, was fascinated. It struck me as interesting that children, in their innocence of cancer and death, know how to respond more appropriately than adults. My baldness was now something exotic and beautiful to him rather than something to be hidden or feared. I agree. I loved my head with the painting but I also love it without the painting. Although I welcome the return of my hair, I will very much miss my head as it is now. This was in total contrast to my initial fears. I believe that when you have determination to make the best of something, even cancer, all kinds of possibilities, including art, can emerge."

photograph by Clay Patrick McBride

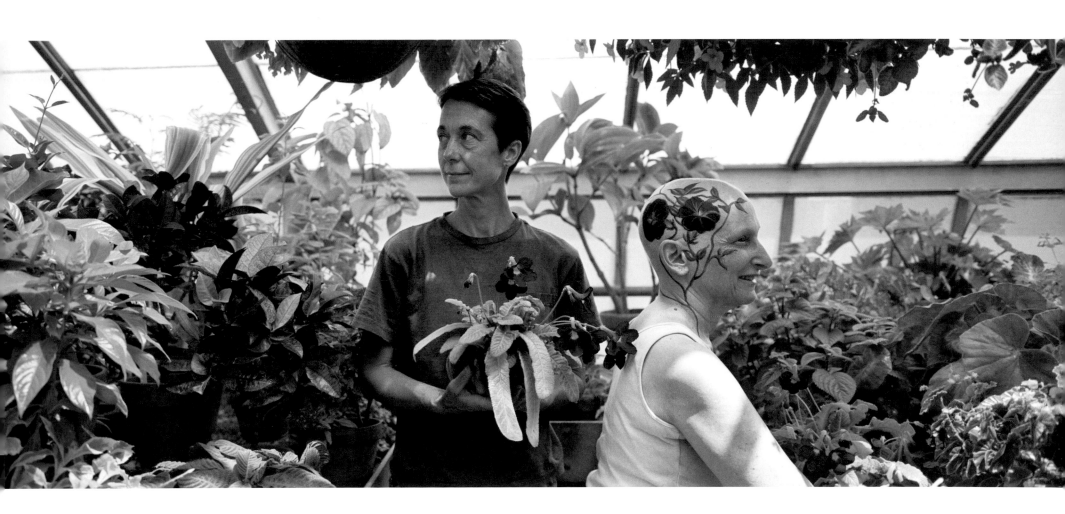

TRACY KAZAN
age 35, stay-at-home mom

"I have three children: Adina who is seven, Joshua, four, and the baby, Victoria, who is fourteen months. When I first told Adina and Joshua I had cancer, Adina asked a lot of questions and handled it beautifully. I didn't tell them that I would lose my hair until a month later. I didn't want to bring it up until it was imminent. Adina was upset but not for the reason we thought. She was distraught about what her friends and the people at school would say. So we talked it out and I made a promise that I would never go out of the house without something on my head. Then I put on a hat for her and showed her how I'd look and I put on a scarf so she saw it wouldn't be bad.

I also asked a friend who had had cancer to come over and show Adina pictures of how she had looked bald. Adina could see that my friend's hair had grown back and it was beautiful and shiny and long. Adina could see that things would get back to normal.

My friends gave me a hat shower which helped. A hat shower is just like a baby shower only you bring hats. They don't have to be store-bought. They can be old baseball caps your friends have lying around. Anything. A bandanna. After the shower, I had about forty hats. I could open the closet and look at them and say, Hey, which one will I put on today? I could see how many people care and love me and that's really nice. I also knew who gave me what hat. When your friends give you hats, it's like they're with you. On days I was feeling impatient, I'd pick up my friend Alana's hat and put it on because she's very patient. Another friend is very organized. If I was feeling disorganized, I'd pick up her hat. Now my kids laugh and joke about the whole thing. They call me 'Baldy Mommy' – nothing's sacred in my house."

photograph by Melissa Ann Pinney

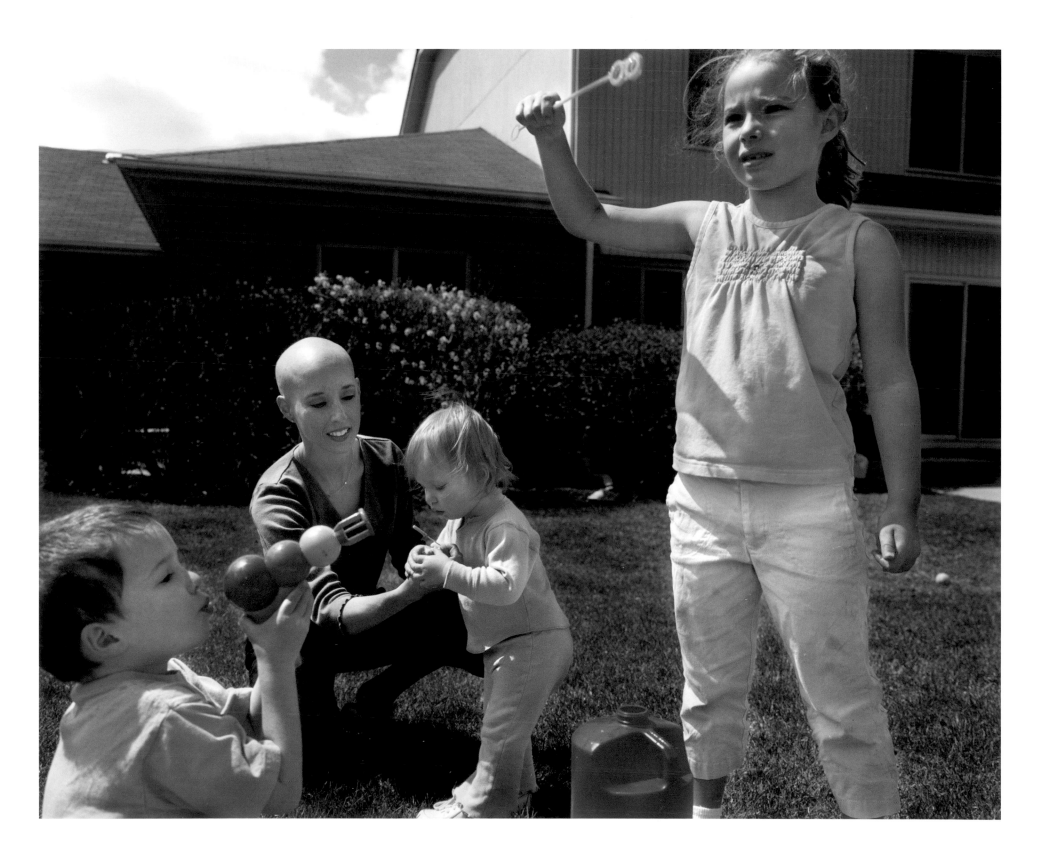

JUSTICE BARBARA PARIENTE
age 55, florida state supreme court justice

"I was tired of feeling hot and uncomfortable in my wigs. I decided to go bare-headed. I had felt I was hiding the real me. I had been worried about people's reaction but realized that I could show everyone that undergoing chemo is not shameful or terrible; it's an affirmation of life, of our willingness to do what is necessary to ensure good health. Women do not have to feel this is something to hide.

Not to say I'm a type of Superwoman, but if your work is not physically arduous, it can have positive benefits. It keeps your mind off what ifs and worries. It's been therapeutic for me. There are a lot more women doing it than commonly known."

(from Justice Pariente's personal diaries and *The Palm Beach Post*)

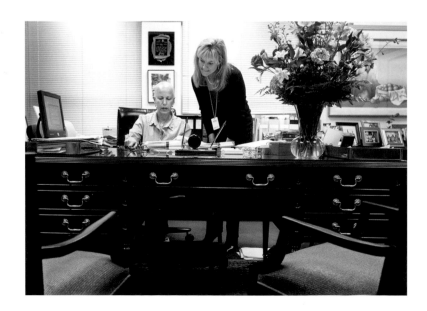

46-

photograph by Jennifer Podis

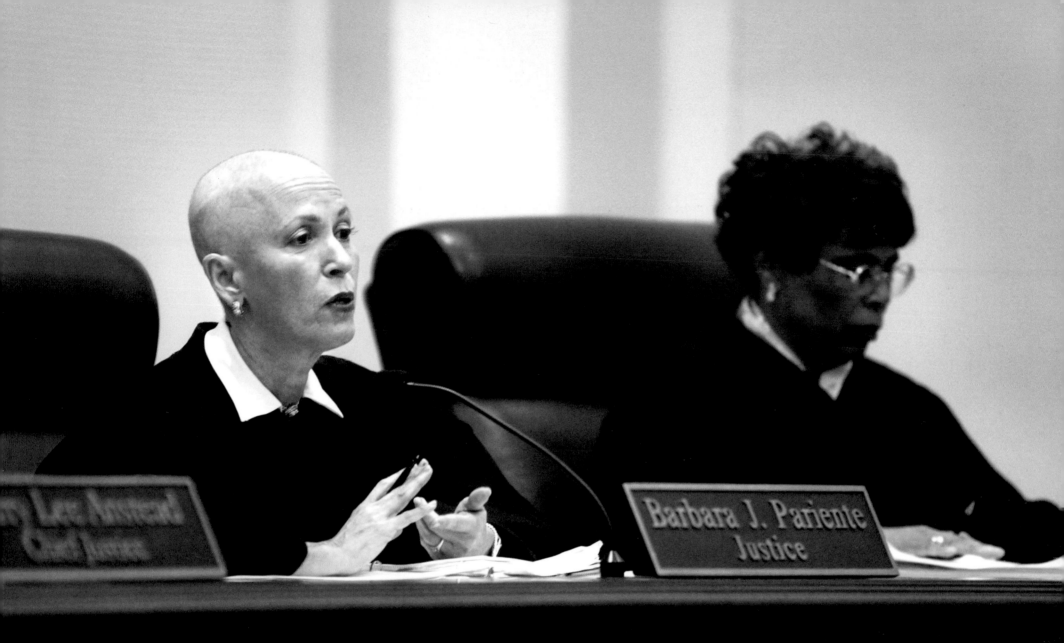

BEVERLY WITHERSPOON
age 60, rides shotgun in husband's rig

"After my second treatment, my husband picked me up in his rig and said, 'Honey, we're going to California.' So I rode with him, put a scarf on, tied it back and didn't take that scarf off for three whole days. I felt nauseous just thinking about my hair falling out. My husband said, 'Honey, we're stopping at the Flying J.' So we stopped and went into a tiny trucker's shower and I took off all my clothes and thought to myself that this was sure a new adventure. Then he took these big scissors (the kind with the big, orange handles) and he held each clump of hair and cut it off. I looked in the mirror and there was this new sight and he said, 'Honey, you look adorable.'

That's not all. A few weeks later, I was watching him comb his hair and I said, 'Honey, can I do that?' So he knelt down in front of me and I began brushing his hair. He leaned over and started kissing my chest where my breast used to be and said, 'You know, we have to be nice to this little tittie (he calls them titties) and give it just as much attention. Know why? Because this little tittie gave her life for you.' Isn't that precious?"

photograph by Thia Konig

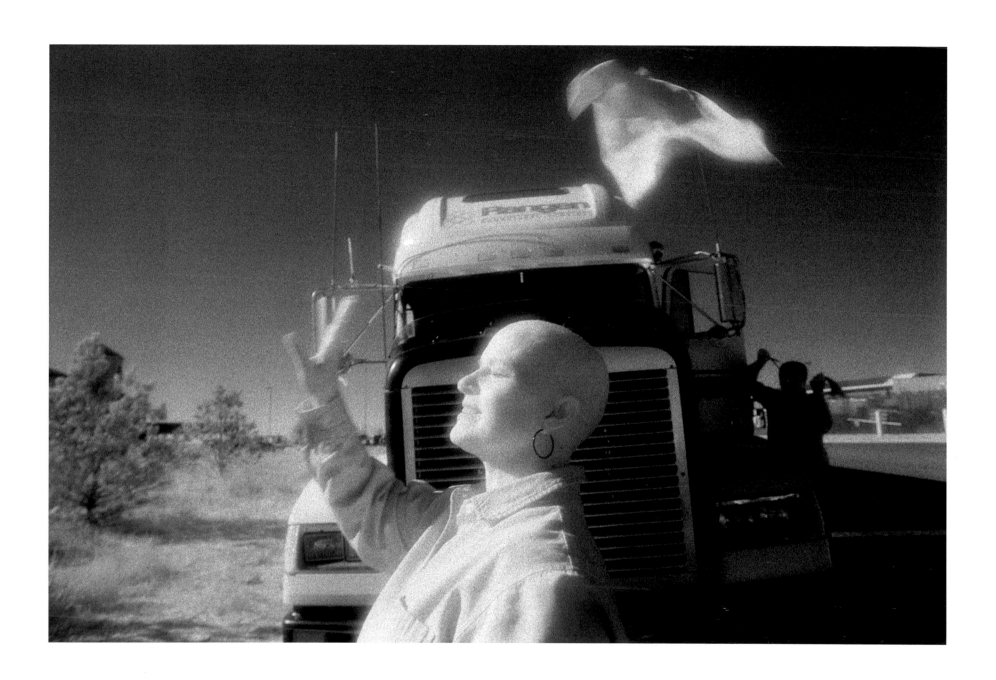

JULIA CHESSER
age 36, communications analyst

"The thing that helped me a lot was being open about it. I had a monthly newsletter going on the Internet. I'd send out upbeat e-mails and updates like, 'Today I finished chemo,' or 'I don't glow yet but after a few more times, watch out, I might.'

My friends would send e-mails back. Their notes helped me keep going and they helped me be positive, knowing how many people were out there trying to help. I don't know how many prayer lists I'm on. I told my aunt, 'God's got to be sick of hearing my name.'"

photograph by Eddie Adams

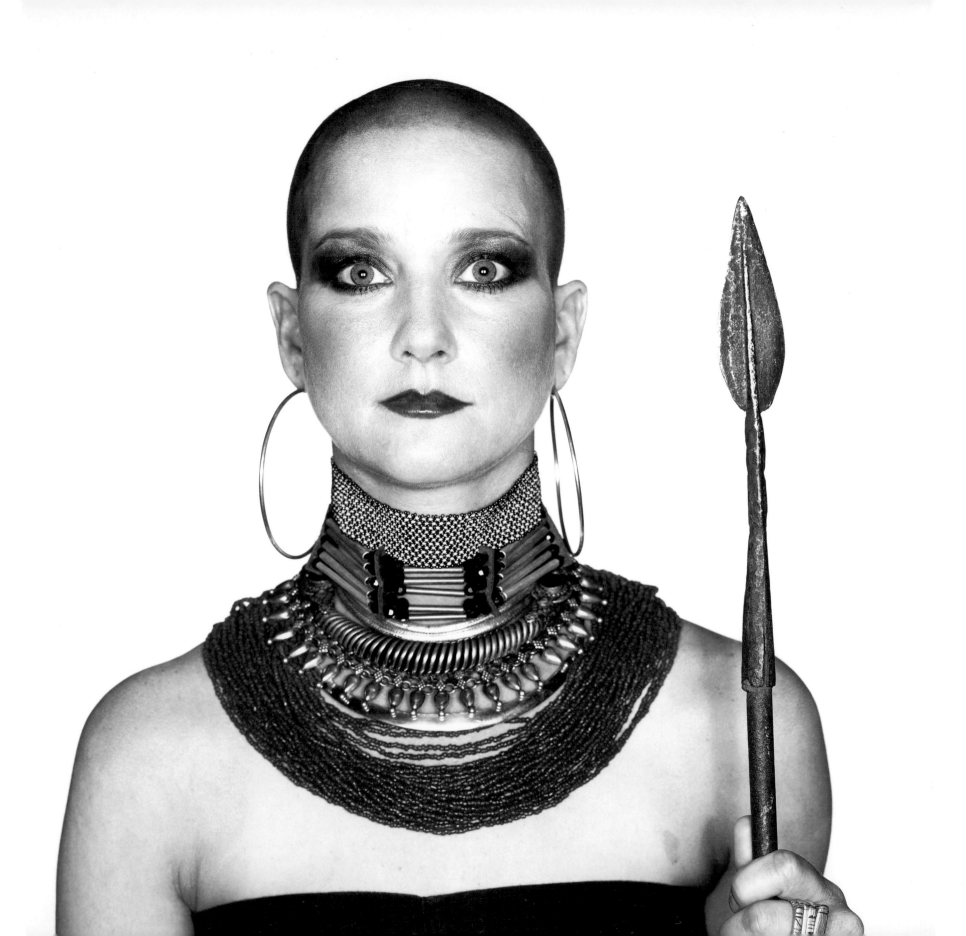

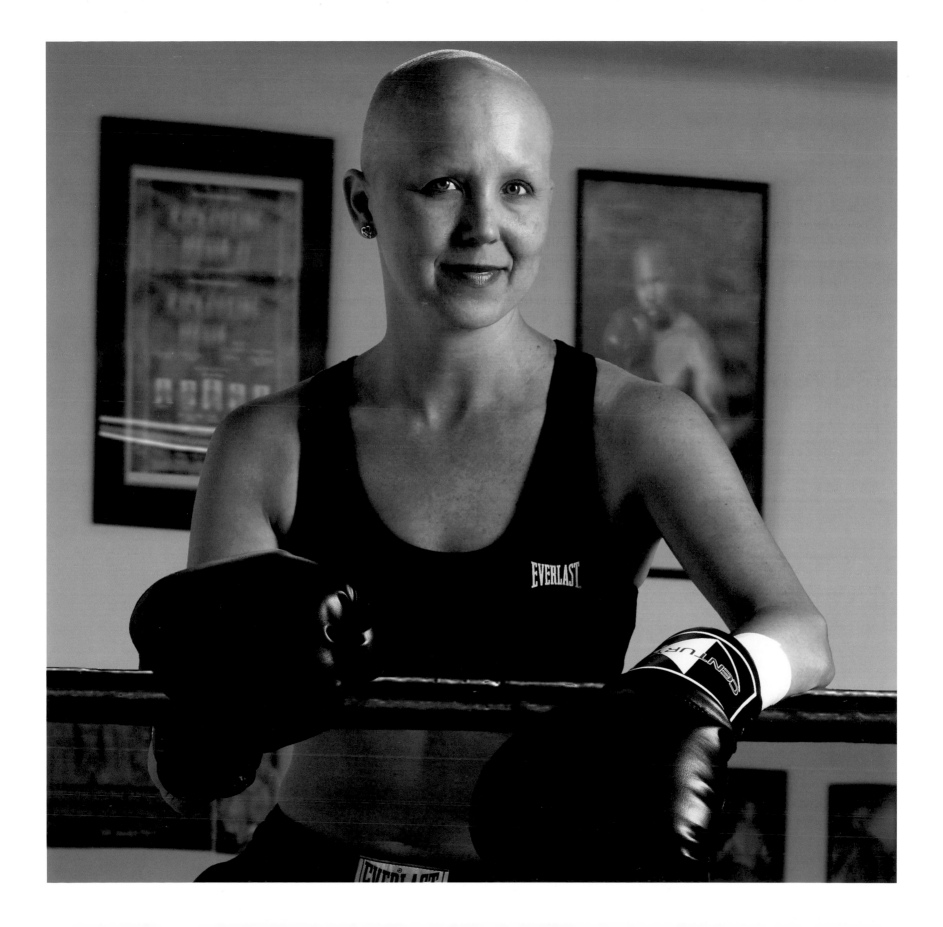

KAREN KEEFER
age 43, ophthalmology administrator

"After I buzzed off my hair, I went upstairs to my bedroom with my husband. I didn't know what to do. Should I put on one of those wigs? Do I put on one of those silly nightcaps they give you? Would I wear one of those caps when I made love to this man? I remember going to my bedroom wearing the cap and there he was and I remember feeling that feeling you have the first time you show your body to a man, not the exciting part but the vulnerable part, like once he sees me exposed, will he still accept me? I mean, here I am, madly in love with this man and somehow afraid of his reaction to my body; feeling that somehow it would change everything about our intimacy.

It's so silly but it took me a week before I felt comfortable with it. It wasn't him, it was me. And then he shaved my head right down to being bald and I suddenly felt it was fun and that it was going to be okay and that he would still see me in the same way he always saw me. Now we'll be in bed together and he'll rub my head or if I get some peach fuzz and it's not even, he'll shave it."

photograph by Barry Goldstein

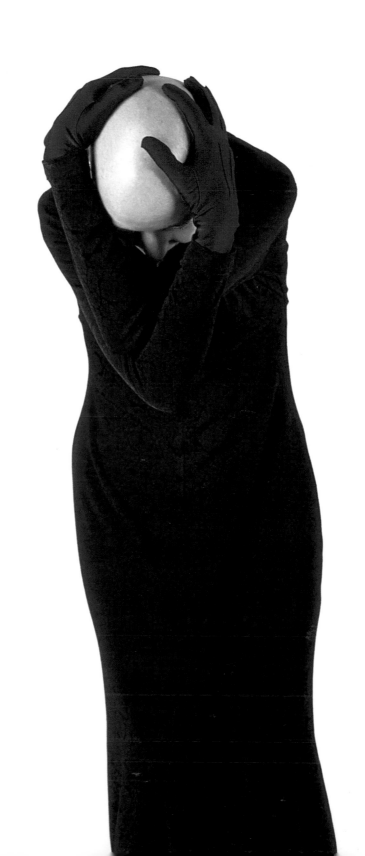

MARCIA REID MARSTED
age 61, writer / photographer

"Lots of people thought I was really brave. But I didn't think I was really brave. I was actually feeling a little guilty about it. Someone said that it was just that I didn't let things bother me. If people see you're dealing with it well, then they call you brave. It's their word for a compliment. But it's not the right word. Tough is a better word.

No one should have the 'Why me?' attitude. It's a totally useless question. You're never going to get the answer and all it's going to do is bother you. It's better to try to live as normal a life as possible. And maybe if you get cancer, maybe you can do something good with it, something that would be helpful to other people or to yourself or your future. Maybe it's more of a wake-up call than a punishment."

photograph by Joyce Tenneson

MICHELLE DAVIS
age 40, pet sitter / animal activist

"I met one of my closest friends while working at an animal hospital. She was a client there. She came in and we hit it off immediately. We both loved dogs, especially cocker spaniels. It turned out we had other things in common. Six months into my treatment, she found out she had cancer, too. We laugh about it now. She says she got sick so that I wouldn't have to go through it alone.

I'm proud that I have been so emotionally strong. I used to think of myself as fragile and delicate but I'm not. I feel if I survived this, I can do anything. The small stuff is just that, small. Petty details won't bother me so much in the future. The big picture is important."

photograph by Harry Langdon

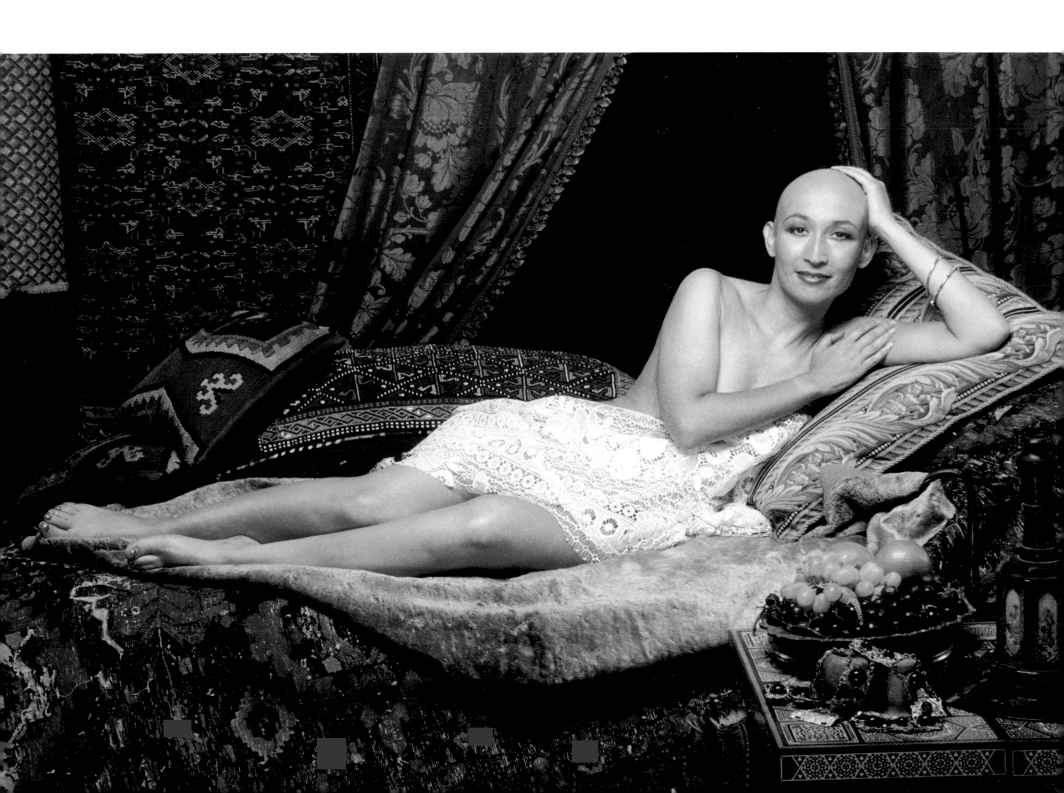

DIANE BAGLEY
age 47, hospital housekeeping

"I felt ugly, lonely, sad, and embarrassed when I first lost my hair. I still feel that way now. Every woman should have hair. I even told the doctor I didn't want to have treatment because I didn't want to lose my hair. He said, 'Okay Diane, you just go home and think about it. Do you want to go through treatment and get better and have your hair grow back, or do you just want to keep your hair?' Even though my friends tell me I look good, I still don't believe my hair will ever grow back."

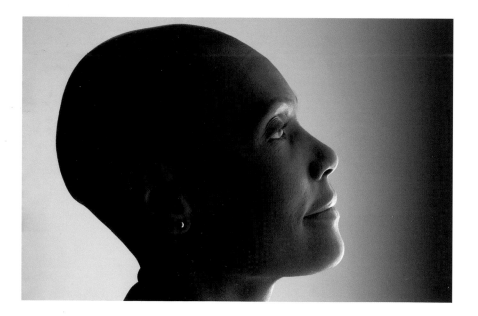

photograph by Jay Maisel

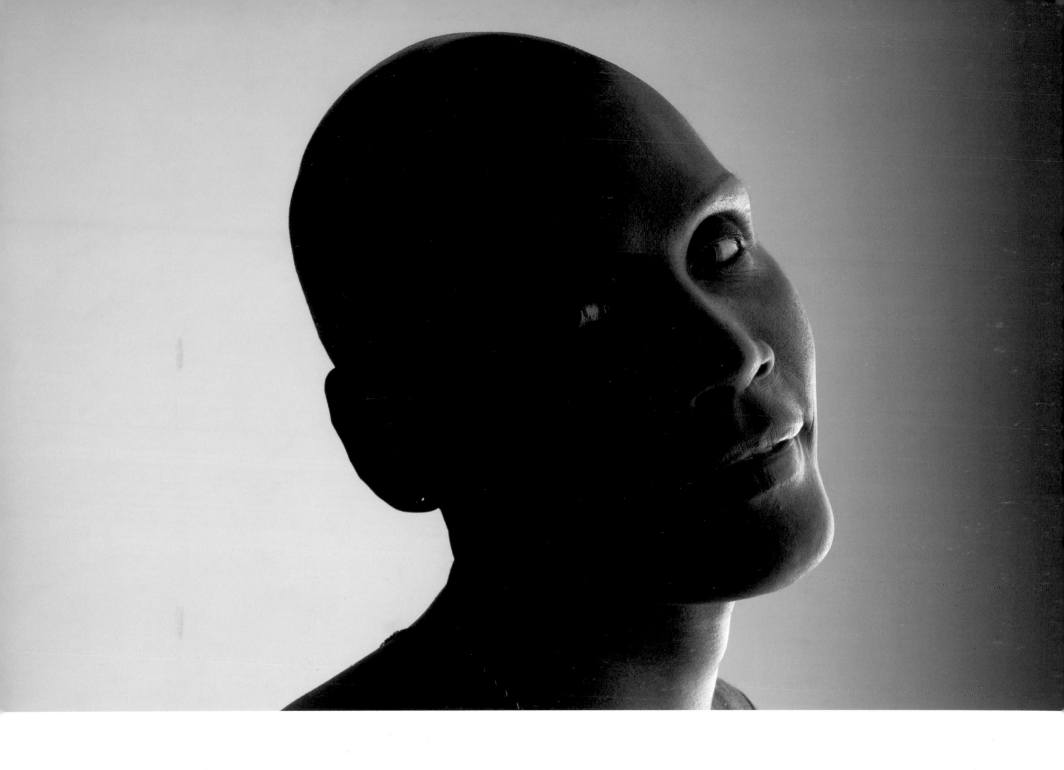

SUE LABONTE
age 39, electrical engineer

"My son started playing hockey when he was four. My husband was the helping coach and I was there as a hockey mom. At the end of the season all the coaches got together to have a coach's game and it looked like a blast. So I started to play.

I landed on the most hilarious team. It was a ball of laughs in the locker room and on the bench and on the ice. I got hooked, although there are plenty of times that I'd think, Oh for a sport where I could just wear cleats and sneakers. Please get me off this thin blade of steel! It was a lot more fun than frustrating, though.

After the diagnosis, I told my team I'd be playing through the season but I didn't know about the next season. A lot of the nurses at Dana Farber (in Boston) thought that the more physical you are the more you can tolerate chemo. My oncologist thought it was okay. So I kept playing.

Sometimes after I'd get treatment, I'd feel it in my quads and bones and I'd think Wow, you had a hell of an exercise yesterday and then I'd remember that it was only the chemo. Other times, you'd feel like you'd gotten crunched, like you'd been hit the day before or beaten up. But as soon as I'd get to my locker and lace up my skates, get my pads on and step out on the ice, I wouldn't feel a thing; I'd grab my stick and take a shot!"

photograph by Ira Wyman

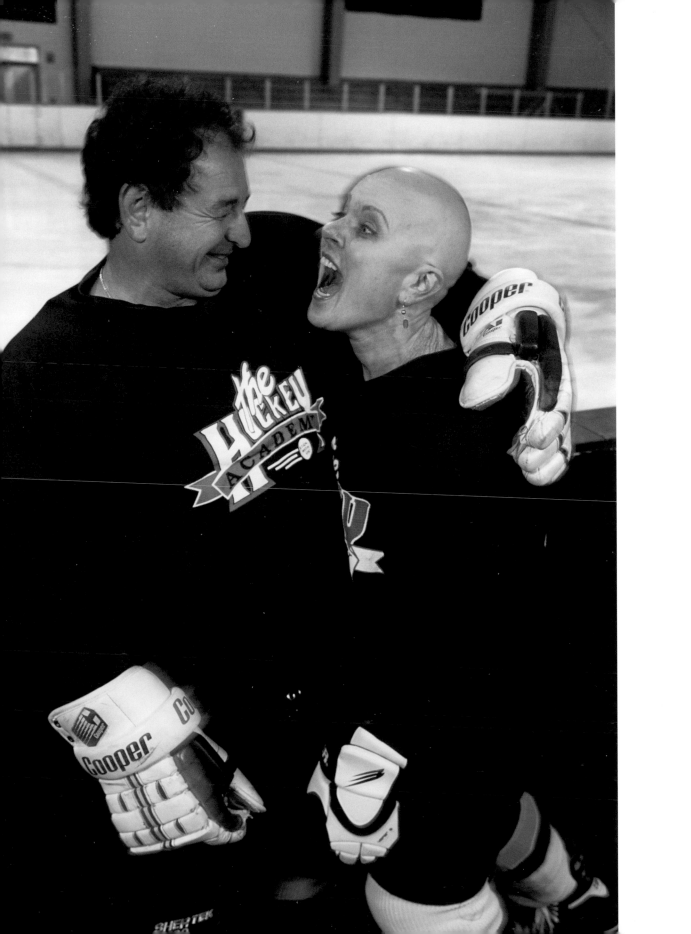

PAM CLERIHAN
age 58, artist

"When something happens to someone you love and it changes their physical appearance, it's hard. When you see that person, you try not to show any emotion because you don't want to hurt or embarrass them. When I knew I was going to lose my hair, my first concern was that my family and friends and neighbors would look at me and feel ill-at-ease.

I'd heard someplace about a lady who had a party when she cut off her hair so I invited everyone I knew including my hairdresser. We had champagne and wine and I sat in a chair in front of them. [Here, she tears up, remembering.] Sorry, I'm kind of weepy today. Anyway, the hairdresser shaved it off. I found out I had a perfectly shaped head.

After the party, from that moment on, there wasn't any 'Oh-look-at-her...' look. We all lost my hair together."

photograph by Michael Childers

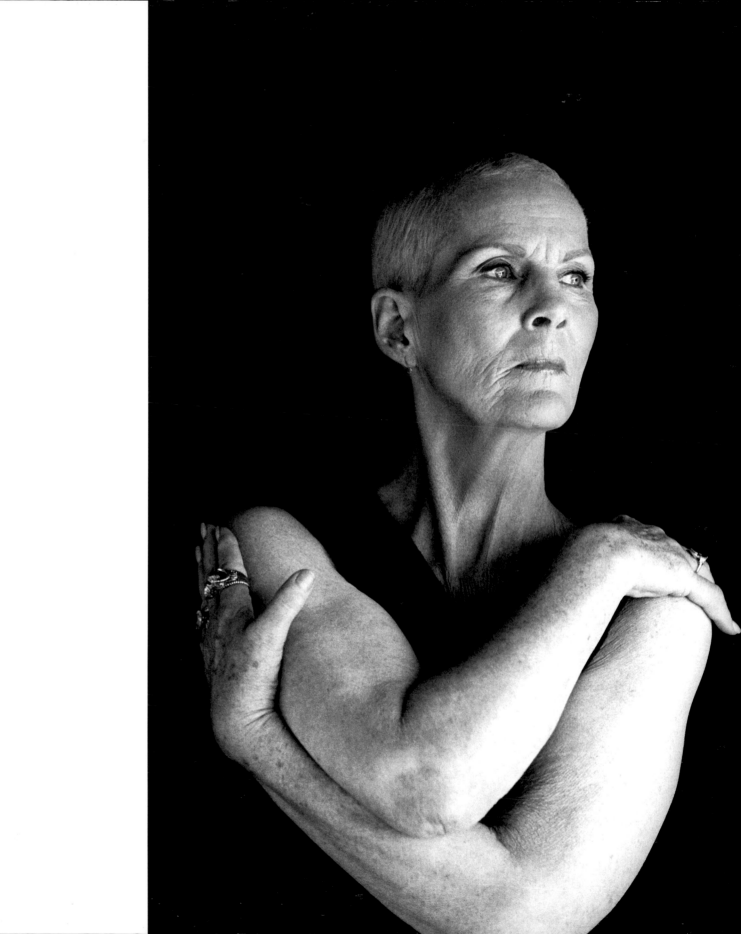

SHARON FRYDA BLYNN
age 32, writer / model

"Just yesterday these three guys were on the train sitting next to me and I could hear them saying all kinds of stupid stuff about my lack of hair. I happened to be wearing combat boots because they're the only boots I have that are good for snowy weather and the cold. I guess I might have looked like some skinhead which is funny because I'm a really nice Jewish girl.

They said something, I forget what, and then one of them said as he was getting off the train, 'God forgive me if this woman has cancer.' I looked at him and said, 'Well, I used to.' And he said, 'Oh, shit.' And he got off the train and the doors closed.

I was thinking just for that brief second, I pushed a button in him so that he and his friends might not do that again. The next time they see a bald woman, they might not make fun of her. They might see her and smile and say, 'You look beautiful today,' and make her feel better."

photograph by Tracy Cwick

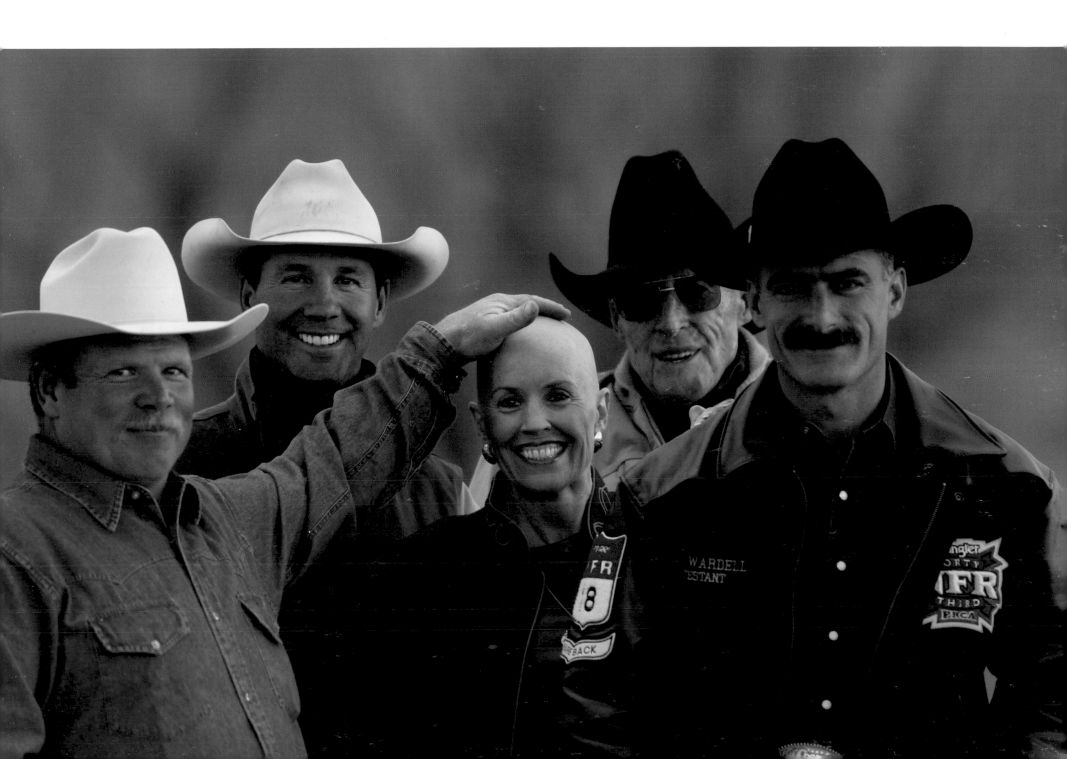

SUSAN MASTONDREA

age 61, medical / surgical buyer

"I live in New York, in Little Italy, and I went into an Italian restaurant in my neighborhood after all my hair fell out. The waitresses there know me and they hadn't seen me for a while so they came up and said, 'What the hell happened to you?' And I told them and they said, 'You have to speak with Barbara, one of our waitresses. A weird thing is happening to her. She had a perfect mammogram and they told her everything was fine but she has a lump above the breast tissue.' They plopped Barbara down in front of me and she was so afraid for her life that she ran out of the restaurant, crying.

Of course, Italians are very dramatic – I can say that because I'm Italian – so they ran out after her. I followed as well and said, 'Barbara, look, this is your life. You've got to go back to the doctor and demand to have a sonogram. You have to make sure. You must.' We left it at that.

A couple of weeks passed. I wondered what had happened. Last Sunday I went back to the restaurant and Barbara was there and she sat down at my table and told me what had happened. 'You're my angel,' she said. 'I went to the doctors the following day and demanded the sonogram. They found breast cancer and now I'm having it taken care of.'

I'm a Buddhist who chants *nam myoho renge kyo* and I believe that I was in that restaurant at the crucial moment to help this stranger with a uniquely similar complaint. My determination today is to help others with cancer. Barbara was my answer to a prayer as I was an answer to her prayer. These moments are what make life beautiful between people."

photograph by Antonin Kratchovil –VII

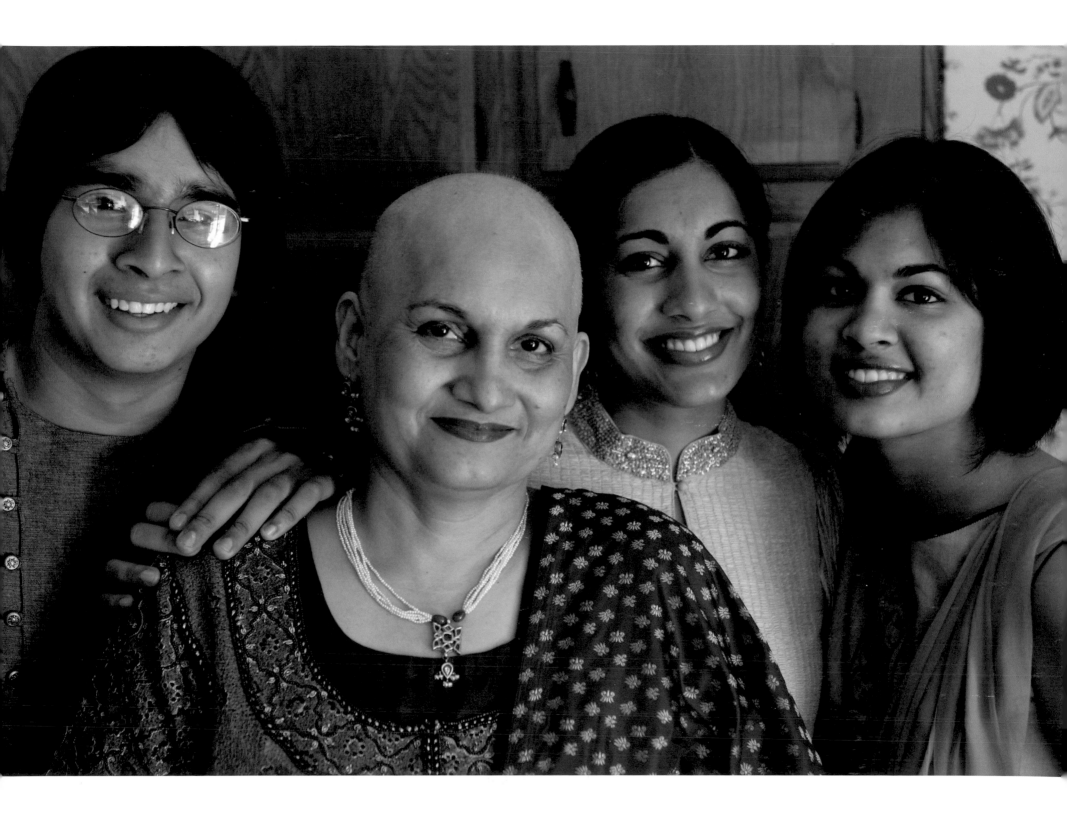

BETTE CROUSE

age 76, native american rights activist, seneca nation

"Before modern medicine, we always had herbs and ways of treating people in the Seneca Nation. We actually had people who would analyze your dreams and tell you what you needed for your particular problem. We had dream analysis long before Freud.

Today, as a rule, when someone has cancer, a member of the Seneca Nation submits herself to modern medicine. In addition, we use the traditional customs for effecting a cure. One such tradition is that someone burns Indian tobacco to send a prayer for your recovery.

I'm not aware of any specific tradition that involves American Indian women and their hair. I was always proud of my hair. It was thick and easy to wear. I never curled or set my hair or did anything like that with it. After I got cancer, I decided I wasn't going to buy a wig. To get a good one, they are very, very expensive. I probably wouldn't have worn one in the summer anyway, it's so hot – but a wig costs so much it would be a shame to spend all that money when you could feed a large number of homeless people instead."

photograph by Karen Ballard

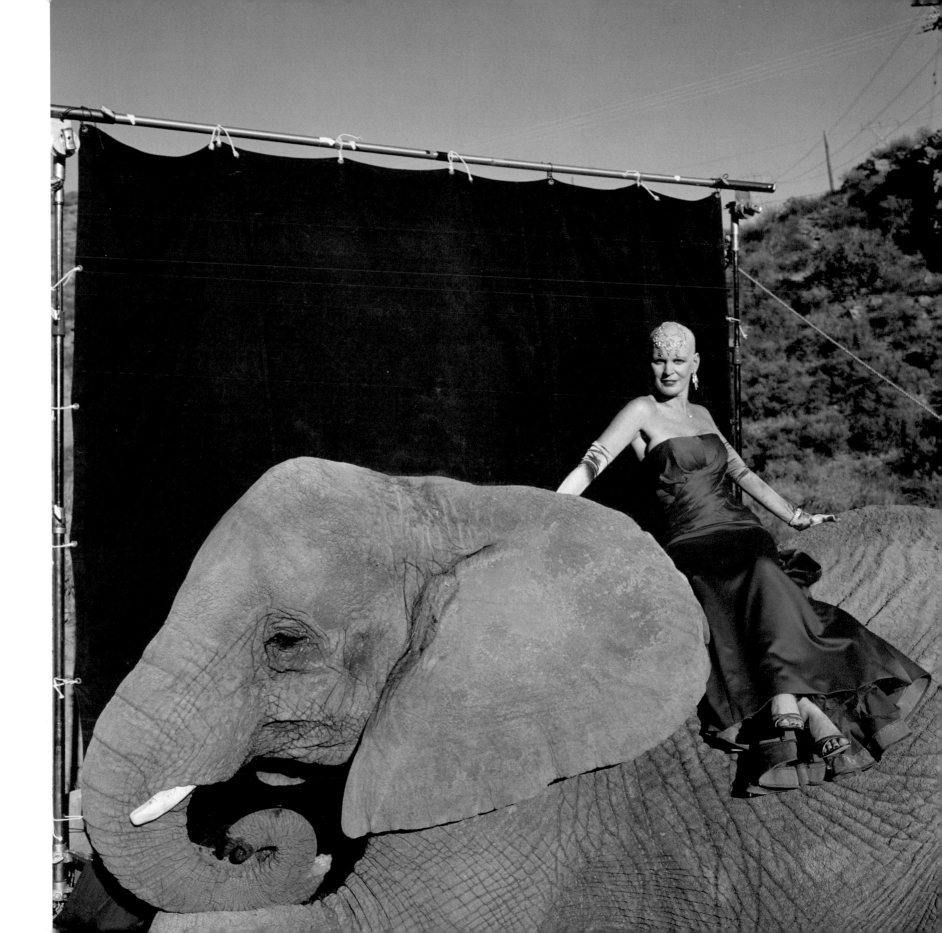

HARRIET KIMBLE WYRE

age 64, psychologist / writer

"Each of our cancers will have our own signature, not just in terms of the lab report, but psychologically. How we handle it is usually how we've handled our lives up until this point. We don't change the way we handle adversity when we get sick. If we've been depressive, we'll probably get depressed. If we chose the pathway of denial, we'll probably continue along that path. If we're obsessive, we'll probably obsess. Now there can be some value to each of those paths if it isn't carried too far. Getting cancer *is* depressing, and grieving is important, but there is also such a thing as some healthy denial. An obsessive style can help us rigorously pursue Internet research about treatment options and lifestyle changes. So it helps to be conscious about the path we choose.

However we deal with it, cancer offers a big chance to wake up and show up on this planet and experience the journey fully. This isn't just a medical thing, it's a journey of much deeper magnitude. For me it's really opening up all my pores to the present moment, even wider than I ever dreamed possible."

photograph by Gerd Ludwig

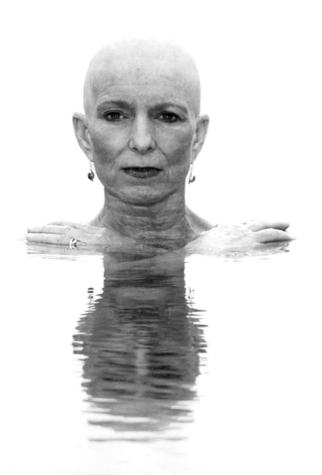

JULIE GOISET
age 28, massage therapist

"Right now I'm bald and I should be bald. It's what you have to do to go through treatment. So accept it. And remember it. Chemotherapy is stressful enough, you shouldn't have to worry about what other people are going to say. Most people are fine with it. You do get some weird looks though, like, 'Oh my God, what's wrong with her?' And that's scary because I've always wanted to be accepted by everyone and that definitely makes me stand out.

Stay strong. There were many times that I thought I wasn't going to make it. I always wanted to give up but I didn't and I'm glad I didn't. I made it through in one piece. A lot of the time I was afraid. I let my mind go to the fear and that made it worse than it really was. It's true when people say 'Try to think positive.' It really does help.

Also take it easy. Don't push yourself. This is a time that you should take for yourself and heal."

photograph by Greg Gorman

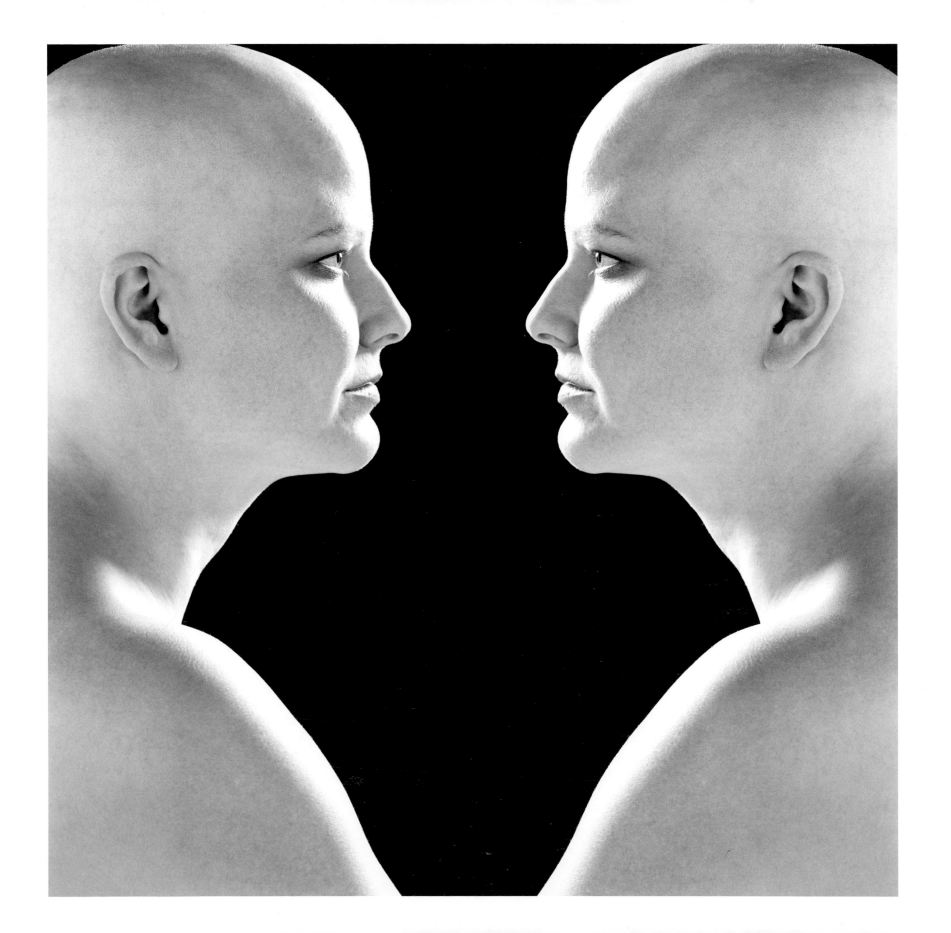

STEFANIE MARCUS
age 29, real estate agent / mother

"My husband and I have both grown up here in Houston. But we are both country people. We love the country and farm animals and everyone being friendly to each other and all that. We've always wanted to move out of the city but we've been kind of stuck primarily because we grew up here and my husband's job is here.

After we found out I had cancer, we said 'Why are we doing this, we're not happy here?' Now our house is on the market, someone has bought it, we're moving to a place that doesn't have a McDonald's or a Wal-Mart. It doesn't even have a stoplight, only a flashing light and a stop sign. For years we've wanted to do it. It took me getting sick to get us strong enough to do it. We tell our friends, life is too short, we want to be happy living it!"

photograph by David Black

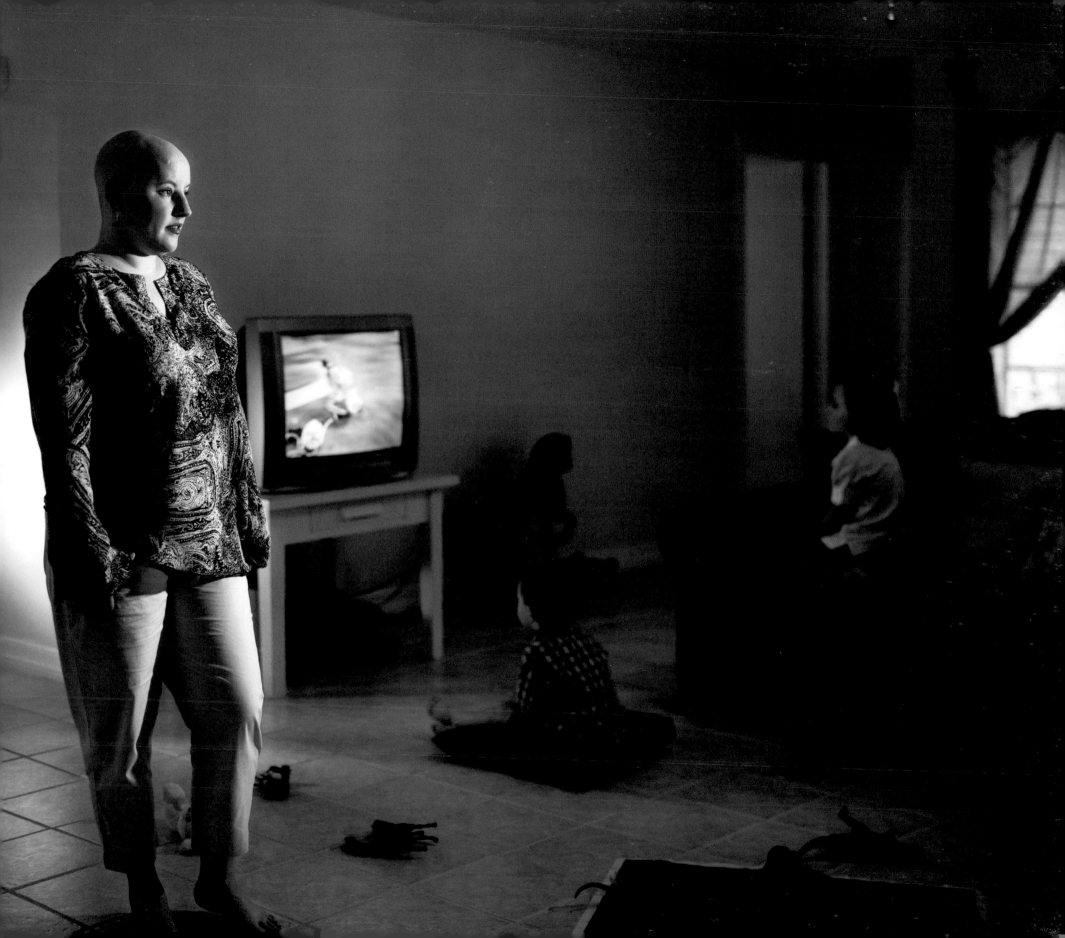

JOY ORDUNA LORENZANNA
age 43, academic advisor / health-care professional

"Western Costume is one of the biggest costume houses in Hollywood. They have costumed films like *Gone With the Wind, The Wizard of Oz, Titanic, Chicago,* and just about any other period film you can think of. I got permission to wear whatever I wanted from all the clothes in their huge, airport-sized warehouse. It was like I was playing dress-up and my mother's closet was a half-a-mile long. Every employee stopped working on whatever it was that they were working on and concentrated on me.

When we started to shoot, suddenly a mysterious man walked up to me and he told me I was beautiful but I needed some jewelry. I had no idea who he was or what was going on or why he was interrupting. He handed me a velvet box and inside the box, were the most beautiful pearls I've ever seen! Pearls, I later found out, that cost $200,000. They were the same pearls that J.Lo wore at the 2003 Oscars. The man in the suit was Garrett Keller from Harry Winston's. Bobi Garland, the head of the library at Western, had arranged the whole thing to surprise me. I couldn't believe it! Then I looked around the warehouse and saw guards with their eyes glued to the pearls around my neck and it finally sunk in.

This picture is really my Oscar because for that one day, I was treated like a star. Who ever gets a chance to do that?"

photograph by Michael Garland

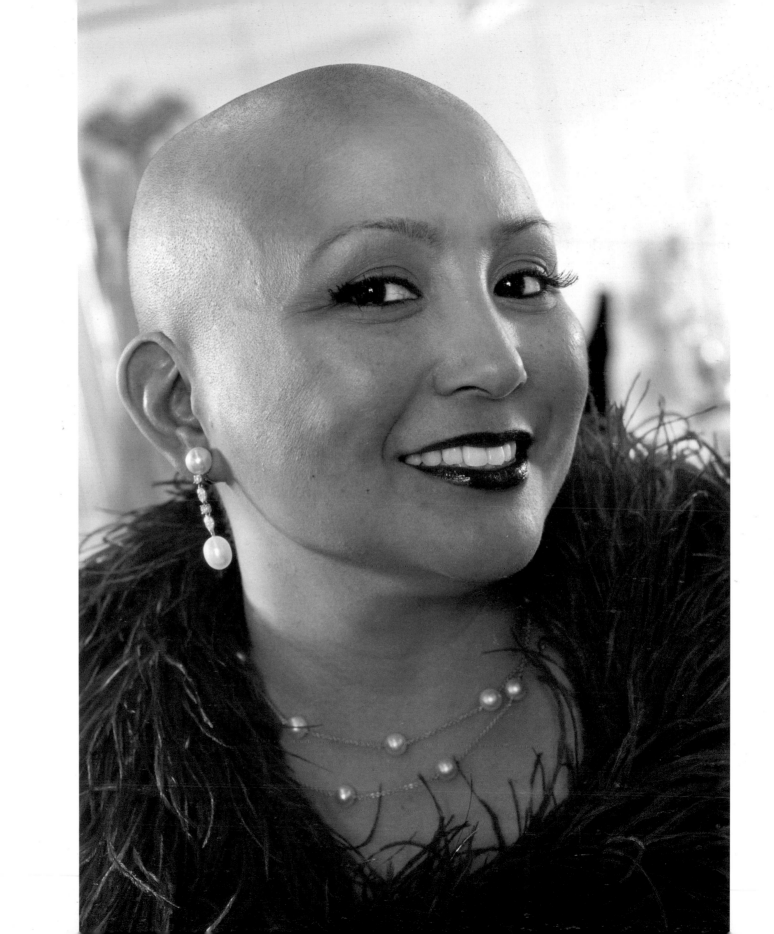

LINELL COMEAUX CHAMPAGNE
age 50, retail

"Before treatment I had a hard time with the not knowing. The not knowing is much worse than the knowing. You need to educate yourself as much as you can. If you can't do it yourself, get a close friend to. Educating yourself helps you get to the next stage which is to tell yourself that you can battle it. Look at all the people out there who have already done it.

My husband is very funny. I knew he was a good man but you never know how good someone is until something like this happens. When he heard, he immediately told me he couldn't imagine life without me. We both cried. We had some moments but then we immediately agreed that we couldn't change because of the diagnosis, we were going to go on and continue to be 'us.' Now, whenever he has the opportunity, he describes us to whoever will listen: 'We've got two bald heads and when we put them together we look like a woman with a low-cut blouse.' "

photograph by Debbie Fleming Caffery